Practical Fracture Treatment

Ronald McRae FRCS (Eng) FRCS (Glas) AIMBI

Formerly Consultant Orthopaedic Surgeon, Southern General Hospital, Glasgow, UK

Max Esser FRCS Ed FRCS Ed (Orth) FRACS (Orth)

Orthopaedic Surgeon, Alfred Hospital, Melbourne; Department of Trauma Surgery, Alfred Hospital, Monash University, Melbourne; Cabrini Hospital, Melbourne, Australia

Original drawings by Ronald McRae

FIFTH EDITION

ELSEVIER
CHURCHILL
LIVINGSTONE

EDINBURGH   LONDON   NEW YORK   OXFORD   PHILADELPHIA   ST LOUIS   SYDNEY   TORONTO   2008

ELSEVIER
CHURCHILL
LIVINGSTONE

First edition 1981
Second edition 1989
Third edition 1994
Fourth edition 2002
Reprinted 2003 (twice), 2004
Fifth edition 2008

ISBN: 978-0-443-06876-8
 Reprinted2008
International Student Edition: ISBN 978-0-443-06877-5

British Library Cataloguing in Publication Data
A catalogue record for this book is available from the British Library.

Library of Congress Cataloging in Publication Data
A catalog record for this book is available from the Library of Congress.

Note
Knowledge and best practice in this field are constantly changing. As new research and experience broaden our knowledge, changes in practice, treatment and drug therapy may become necessary or appropriate. Readers are advised to check the most current information provided (i) on procedures featured or (ii) by the manufacturer of each product to be administered, to verify the recommended dose or formula, the method and duration of administration, and contraindications. It is the responsibility of the practitioner, relying on their own experience and knowledge of the patient, to make diagnoses, to determine dosages and the best treatment for each individual patient, and to take all appropriate safety precautions. To the fullest extent of the law, neither the Publisher nor the Authors assume any liability for any injury and/or damage to persons or property arising out or related to any use of the material contained in this book.

The Publisher

Printed in China

Practical
Fracture
Treatment

For Elsevier:
Commissioning Editor: Alison Taylor
Development Editor: Kim Benson
Production Manager: Kerrie-Anne Jarvis
Design: George Ajayi

CONTENTS

PREFACE TO THE FIFTH EDITION

As in the previous edition more recent methods of internal fixation in the treatment of many fractures have been included, while the basics of conservative management and plaster cast techniques have been retained. This is considered to be important, particularly in situations where access to the wide variety of implants and imaging equipment required for many internal fixation procedures may be limited.

Several new fracture classifications have been detailed, and in many areas new thoughts on the management of some specific fractures have been reviewed and treatment suggestions modified. An appreciable number of drawings illustrating new implants and the techniques that they involve have been added.

There are also many new radiographs, CT scans and 3-D reconstructions, and in the continued quest to improve the clarity of reproduction, digital enhancements, judicious cropping, and the addition of arrows and dotted lines have been carried out on certain radiographs – or substitutions made.

In this edition a number of references, which have been considered to be of particular value have been included.

We hope that these changes will add to the value of this book.

Ronald McRae, Gourock 2008
Max Esser, Melbourne 2008

Acknowledgements

I wish to acknowledge the help I have had from my colleagues at the Alfred Hospital: in particular Associate Professor Alison Street, Haematologist; Associate Professor Nina Sacharias, Radiologist; Mr Ross Snow, Urologist; and the Audio Visual Department. Mr Greg Malham, Neurosurgeon, Alfred Hospital, and Professor Thomas Kossmann, Department of Trauma Surgery, Alfred Hospital were generous with their advice and comments. My friend and colleague Mr Gary Nattrass, Royal Children's Hospital, Melbourne, once again contributed with valuable suggestions.

My wife Kym and our two children, Nick and Lauren, who were very tolerant and supportive in this project, for which I am grateful.

Once again Kaye Lionello, my secretary, contributed greatly to this edition with multiple e-mails and incalculable patience.

Max Esser, Melbourne 2008

PREFACE TO THE FIRST EDITION

This book has been written primarily for the medical student, and the introductory section assumes little prior knowledge of the subject. *The second part*, which deals with particular fractures, is set in places at a more advanced level; it is hoped that the book will thereby continue to prove of value to the student when he moves to his first casualty or registrar post.

In planning this volume, I have paid particular attention to two points. Firstly, the details of each fracture and a good deal of the introductory section have been arranged in a linear sequence. The material has been divided into small packets of text and illustration in order to facilitate comprehension and learning. These packets have been set out in a logical sequence which in most cases is based on the relative importance of the initial decisions which must be made in a case, and the order in which treatment procedures should be carried out. This format is in a few places restrictive, with an imbalance in the amount of information carried by either text or illustration. This must be accepted because of spatial and subject limitations. Generally, however, text and illustration will be found to complement one another. The text, although of necessity brief, is concise and, it is hoped, to the point.

Secondly, fracture treatment has been given in an uncommon amount of practical detail. As there is such a variety of accepted treatments for even the simplest of fractures, this has the danger of attracting the criticism of being controversial and didactic. This is far from my intention, and I have tried to avoid this in several ways. Firstly, as minor fractures and most children's fractures (together forming the bulk of all fractures) are most frequently treated conservatively, the conservative approach I have employed for these injuries should on the whole receive general approval. Secondly, in the more controversial long bone fractures in adults, and in fractures involving joints, I have on the whole pursued a middle course between the extremes of conservative and surgical management. The methods I have singled out for description are those which I consider safest and most reliable in the hands of the comparatively inexperienced. Where alternative methods appear to me to be equally valid I have generally included these. To conceal my own whims I have not always placed these in the order of personal preference. In consequence, I hope that any offence given by the methods described will be restricted to the most extreme quarters.

R. M.

HOW TO USE THIS BOOK

The basic principle of fractures and their treatment are dealt with in the first part of this book. The AO Classification of fractures (pp 22–24), Trauma scoring (pp 41–44) and the Mangled Extremity Severity Score (pp 51–52) may be noted but do not require detailed study by the undergraduate.

The second part of the book is arranged on a regional basis and may be used as a guide for the handling of specific fractures. Detailed study is not required by the undergraduate, but a superficial reading should consolidate knowledge of the basic principles, and indicate how they are applied in practice.

The following conventions are used in the illustrations and text:

1. Where two sides are shown for comparison, the patient's *right* side is the one affected.
2. As a general rule, when a procedure is being illustrated, the patient is shown for clarification in a lighter tone of grey than the surgeon and his assistants.
3. Where several conditions are described, and only one illustrated, the first mentioned is the one shown, unless followed by the abbreviation 'Illus.'.
4. Most cross references within a chapter are made by quoting the relevant frame number. Elsewhere, page numbers are given.

Abbrevations

A   = anterior
Illus. = illustrated
L   = lateral or left
M   = medial
N   = normal
P   = posterior
R   = right

SECTION

A

General principles

Pathology and healing of fractures

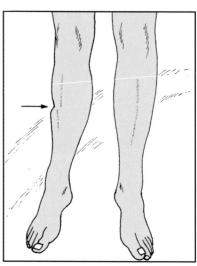

1. Initial definitions: Fracture: A fracture is present when there is loss of continuity in the substance of a bone. The term covers all bony disruptions, ranging from one end of the scale when (1) a bone is broken into many fragments (multifragmentary or comminuted fracture) to (2) hair-line and even microscopic fractures at the other. To the layman the word 'fracture' implies a more severe injury than a simple break in the bone, but in the strict medical sense there is no difference between these terms.

2. Open fractures: All fractures are either *closed or open*. In an open fracture there is a wound in continuity with the fracture, and the potential exists for organisms to enter the fracture site from outside. All open fractures therefore carry the risk of becoming infected. In addition, blood loss from external haemorrhage may be significant. (Note: the term 'compound' is still frequently used to describe a fracture which is open; the term 'simple', to describe a closed fracture, may lead to confusion, and is now largely abandoned.)

3. Closed fracture: In a closed fracture the skin is either intact, or if there are any wounds these are superficial or unrelated to the fracture. So long as the skin is intact, there is no risk of infection from outside. (Blood-borne infection of closed fractures is extremely rare.) Any haemorrhage is internal.

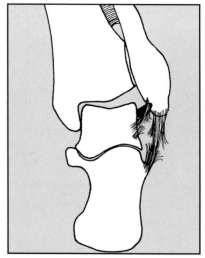

4. Dislocation: In a dislocation there is complete loss of congruity between the articulating surfaces of a joint. The bones taking part in the articulation are displaced relative to one another; e.g. in a dislocated shoulder the head of the humerus loses all contact with the glenoid. In the common anterior dislocation the head of the humerus is displaced anteriorly.

5. Subluxation: In a subluxation, the articulating surfaces of a joint are no longer congruous, but loss of contact is incomplete. The term is often used to describe the early stages in a condition which may proceed to complete dislocation (e.g. in a joint infection or in rheumatoid arthritis).

6. Sprain: A sprain is an incomplete tear of a ligament or complex of ligaments responsible for the stability of a joint; e.g. a sprain of the ankle is a partial tear of the lateral ligament and is not associated with instability (as distinct from a complete tear). The term sprain is also applied to incomplete tears of muscles and tendons.

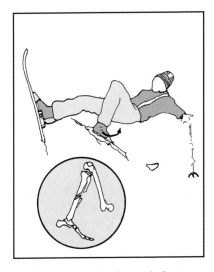

7. Causes of fracture: Direct violence (a): Fractures are caused by the application of stresses which exceed the limits of strength of a bone. Violence is the commonest cause. In the case of *direct violence*, a bone may be fractured by being struck by a moving or falling object, e.g. a fracture of the terminal phalanx of a finger by a hammer blow.

8. Direct violence (b): A bone may also be fractured if *it* forcibly strikes a resistant object. For example, a fall on the point of the elbow may fracture the olecranon.

9. Indirect violence: Very frequently fractures result from indirect violence.
A twisting or bending stress is applied to a bone, and this results in its fracture at some distance from the application of the causal force. For example, a rotational stress applied to the foot may cause a spiral fracture of the tibia. Indirect violence is also the commonest cause of dislocation.

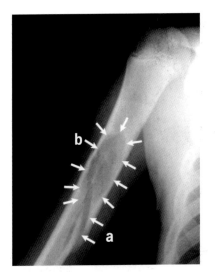

10. Fatigue fractures: Stresses, repeated with excessive frequency to a bone, may result in fracture. This mechanism is often compared with fatigue in metals which break after repeated bending beyond their elastic limit. The commonest of these fractures involves the second metatarsal – the march fracture (so called because of its frequency in army recruits).

11. Pathological fractures (a):
A pathological fracture is one which occurs in an abnormal or diseased bone. If the osseous abnormality reduces the strength of the bone then the force required to produce fracture is reduced, and may even become trivial. For example a secondary tumour deposit may lead to a pathological fracture of the subtrochanteric region of the femur – a common site.

12. Pathological fractures (b): Pathological fractures may also occur at the site of simple tumours, e.g. a fracture of the humerus (a) in a child with a simple bone cyst (b). *The commonest causes of pathological fracture are osteoporosis and osteomalacia.*

13. Fracture patterns and their significance: Hair-line fractures (a): Hair-line fractures result from minimal trauma, i.e. trauma which is just great enough to produce a fracture but not severe enough to produce any significant displacement of the fragments. Such fractures may be (1) incomplete or (2) complete.

14. Hair-line fractures (b): These fractures may be difficult to detect on the radiographs, and where there are reasonable clinical grounds for suspecting a fracture, the rules are quite clear. 1. Additional oblique radiographic projections of the area may be helpful. 2. Do not accept poor quality films. 3. Films repeated after 7–10 days may show the fracture quite clearly (due to decalcification at the fracture site). 4. A CT scan may also help confirm the diagnosis.

15. Hair-line fractures (c): *Stress fractures* are generally hair-line in pattern, and are often not diagnosed with certainty until there is a wisp of subperiosteal callus formation, or increased density at the fracture site some 3–6 weeks after the onset of symptoms. Where strongly suspected an MRI or bone scan may be helpful. Hair-line fractures generally heal rapidly requiring only symptomatic treatment: **but** the scaphoid and femoral neck are notable exceptions.

16. Hair-line fractures (d): Radiograph of upper tibia of an athletic adolescent with a 7-week history of persistent leg pain. Previous radiographs were reported as normal. Note the coned view to obtain optimal detail and the incomplete hair-line fracture revealed by bone sclerosis and subperiosteal callus. A crepe bandage support only was prescribed, and the symptoms settled in a further 6 weeks.

17. Greenstick fractures (a): Greenstick fractures occur in children, but not all children's fractures are of this type. The less brittle bone of the child tends to buckle on the side opposite the causal force. Tearing of the periosteum and of the surrounding soft tissues is often minimal.

18. Greenstick fractures (b): This radiograph illustrates a more severe greenstick fracture of the distal radius and ulna. Note that although there is about 45° of angulation at the fracture site, there is no loss of bony contact in either fracture. The clinical deformity is clearly suggested by the soft-tissue shadow.

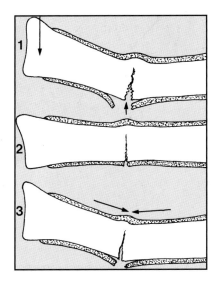

19. Greenstick fractures (c): Reduction of a greenstick fracture is facilitated by the absence of displacement and by the intact tissues on the concavity of the fracture. Angulation may be corrected by supporting the fracture and applying pressure over the distal fragment (1 and 2). The elastic spring of the periosteum may however lead to recurrence of angulation (3). Particular attention must therefore be taken over plaster fixation and after care.

20. Greenstick fractures (d): In the forearm in particular, where angulation inevitably leads to restriction of pronation and supination, some surgeons deliberately overcorrect the initial deformity (1). This tears the periosteum on the other side of the fracture (2). This reduces the risks of secondary angulation (3). Healing in all greenstick fractures is rapid.

21. Simple transverse fractures (a): Transverse fractures run either at right angles to the long axis of a bone (1), or with an obliquity of less than 30°. They may be caused by *direct violence*, when the bone fractures directly beneath the causal force (e.g. the ulna fracturing when warding off a blow (a)). They may also result from *indirect violence* when the bone is subjected to bending stresses by remotely applied force (e.g. a fracture of the forearm bones resulting from a fall on the outstretched hand (b)).

22. Simple transverse fractures (b): The inherent stability of this type of fracture (illustrated by the model on the right) reduces the risks of shortening and displacement. In the tibia, as a result, weight bearing may be permitted at a comparatively early stage. On the other hand, the area of bony contact is small, requiring very strong union before any external support can be discarded. (NB: The term 'simple' used to describe this and the following fractures means that the fracture runs circumferentially round the bone with the formation of only two main fragments.)

23. Simple oblique fractures (a): In an oblique fracture (1) the fracture runs at an oblique angle of 30° or more (O). Such fractures may be caused by (a) direct or (b) indirect violence. In *simple spiral fractures* (2) the line of the fracture curves round the bone in a spiral. Simple spiral fractures result from indirect violence, applied to the bone by twisting (torsional) forces (t).

24. Simple oblique and spiral fractures (b): In spiral fractures, union can be rapid (1) as there is often a large area of bone in contact. In both oblique and spiral fractures, unopposed muscle contraction or premature weight bearing readily lead to shortening, displacement and sometimes loss of bony contact (2). [Note: In the AO Classification of Fractures (see later) simple spiral, oblique and transverse fractures are classified as Type A fractures.]

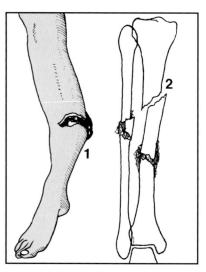

25. In multifragmentary (comminuted) fractures there are more than two fragments. *The spiral wedge fracture* (1) is produced by torsional forces (t), and the *bending wedge fracture* (2) by direct (a) or indirect (b) violence. The fragment (B) is often called a butterfly fragment (because of its shape). With greater violence a *fragmented (comminuted) wedge fracture* (3) results. [All these fractures are in Type B in the AO Classification (see later) and their characteristic is that after reduction there is still bony contact between the main fragments (4)].

26. In multifragmentary complex fractures (a further division of comminuted fractures) there is no contact between the main fragments after reduction. In *complex spiral fractures* (1) there are two or more spiral elements; in *complex segmental fractures (sometimes called double fractures)* (2) there is at least one quite separate complete bone fragment (S). In *complex irregular fractures* (3) the bone lying between the main elements is split into many irregular fragments. [All these fractures are classified as Type C in the AO Classification.]

27. Multifragmentary fractures are generally the result of greater violence than is the case with most simple fractures, and consequently there is an increased risk of damage to neighbouring muscle, blood vessels and skin (1). The fractures tend to be unstable, and delayed union and joint stiffness are common. Segmental fractures are often difficult to reduce by closed methods, and direct exposure may threaten the precarious blood supply to the central segment. Non-union at one level is not uncommon in these fractures (2).

28. Impacted fractures: A fracture is impacted when one fragment is driven into the other (1). Cancellous bone is usually involved and union is often rapid. The *stability* of these fractures varies and is more implied than real. Displacement will occur if the fracture is subjected to deforming forces; e.g. without fixation, impacted femoral neck fractures frequently come adrift (2).

29. Compression (or crush) fractures: Crush fractures occur in cancellous bone which is compressed beyond the limits of tolerance. Common sites are (1) the vertebral bodies (as a result of flexion injuries) and (2) the heels (following falls from a height). If the deformity is accepted, union is invariably rapid. In the spine, if correction is attempted, recurrence is almost invariable.

30. Avulsion fractures (a): An avulsion fracture may be produced by a sudden muscle contraction, the muscle pulling off the portion of bone to which it is attached. Common examples include:
(1) Base of fifth metatarsal (peroneus brevis)
(2) Tibial tuberosity (quadriceps)
(3) Upper pole of patella (quadriceps)
(4) Lesser trochanter (iliopsoas)
(These are all AO Type A fractures.)

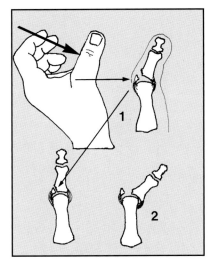

31. Avulsion fractures (b): Avulsion fractures may also result from traction on a ligamentous or capsular attachment: these are often witness of *momentary dislocation;* e.g. (1) an abduction force may avulse the ulnar collateral ligament attachment, with spontaneous reduction. *Late subluxation* (2) is common with this ('gamekeeper's thumb') and other injuries and is especially serious in the case of the spine.

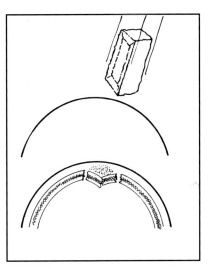

32. Depressed fracture: Depressed fractures occur when a sharply localised blow depresses a segment of cortical bone below the level of the surrounding bone. Although common in skull fractures, this pattern is only rarely found in the limbs. There the tibia in the upper third is probably most frequently affected. Healing is rapid; complications are dependent on the site.

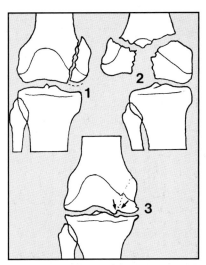

33. Fractures involving the articular surfaces of a joint: In *partial articular fractures* (1) part of the joint surface is involved, but the remainder is intact and solidly connected to the rest of the bone. (AO Type B fracture.) In *complete articular fractures* (2) the articular surface is completely disrupted and separated from the shaft. (AO Type C fracture.) When a fracture involves the articular surfaces, any persisting irregularity may cause secondary osteoarthritis (3). Stiffness is a common complication, and this may be minimised by early mobilisation.

34. Fracture close to a joint: When a fracture lies close to a joint, stiffness may also be a problem due to tethering of neighbouring muscles and tendons by spread of callus from the healing fracture; e.g. in fractures of the femur close to the knee, the quadriceps may become bound down by the callus, resulting in difficulty with knee flexion.

35. Fracture–dislocation: A fracture–dislocation is present when a joint has dislocated and there is in addition a fracture of one of the bony components of the joint. Illustrated is a fracture–dislocation of the shoulder, where there is an anterior dislocation with a fracture of the neck of the humerus. Injuries of this kind may be difficult to reduce and may be unstable. Stiffness and avascular necrosis are two common complications.

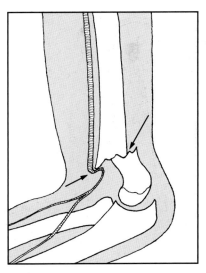

36. Complicated fractures: A fracture is described as complicated if there is accompanying damage to major neighbouring structures. The diagram is of a complicated supracondylar fracture of the humerus. (Such an injury might also be described as a supracondylar fracture complicated by damage to the brachial artery.)

37. Describing the level of a fracture (a): *The anatomical divisions* of a long bone include the epiphysis (E), the epiphyseal plate (EP), and the diaphysis or shaft (D). Between the latter two is the metaphysis (M). A fracture may be described as lying within these divisions, or involving a distinct anatomical part; e.g. (A) = fracture of the tibial diaphysis; (B) = fracture of the femoral neck; (C) = fracture of the greater trochanter; (F) = supracondylar fracture of the femur.

38. Describing the level of a fracture (b): For descriptive purposes a bone may be divided arbitrarily into thirds. In this way (A) = fracture of the mid third of the femur; (B) = fracture of the femur in the distal third; (C) = fracture of the femur at the junction of the middle and distal thirds. The level of a fracture in some cases may be made quite clear by an eponym; e.g. a Colles fracture (D) involves the radius, and occurs within an inch (2.5 cm) of the wrist.

39. Describing the level of a fracture (c): *In AO terminology*, long bones are divided into three unequal segments: *a proximal segment* (1), a central *diaphyseal segment* (2), and a *distal segment* (3). The boundaries between these segments are obtained by erecting squares (S) which accommodate the widest part of the bone ends; in the special case of the femur the diaphysis is described as commencing at the distal border of the lesser trochanter.

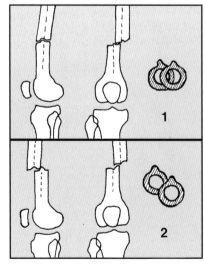

40. Describing the deformity: If there is no deformity, i.e. if the violence which has produced the fracture has been insufficient to cause any movement of the bone ends relative to one another, then the fracture is said to be in anatomical position. Similarly, if a perfect position has been achieved after manipulation of a fracture, it may be described as being in anatomical position.

41. Displacement (a): Displacement (or translation) is present if the bone ends have shifted relative to one another. The direction of displacement is described in terms of movement of the distal fragment. For example, in these fractures of the femoral shaft at the junction of the middle and distal thirds there is (1) no displacement, (2) lateral displacement, (3) posterior displacement, (4) both lateral and posterior displacement.

42. Displacement (b): Apart from the direction of displacement, the degree must be considered. A rough estimate is usually made of the percentage of the fracture surfaces in contact; e.g. (1) 50% bony apposition (2) 25% bony apposition. Good bony apposition encourages stability and union.

84. Growth disturbances (a): If growth is arrested over part of the epiphyseal plate only, there will be progressive angulatory deformity affecting the axis of movement of the related joint. There will be a little overall shortening. This radiograph shows the tilting of the plane of the ankle joint which occurred in the last case, with deformity of the foot and ankle. In the elbow, injuries of this type may lead to cubitus varus or valgus.

85. Growth disturbances (b): If the whole epiphyseal plate is affected, growth will be arrested, leading to greater shortening of the bone. The final result will depend on the age at which epiphyseal arrest occurred, and the epiphysis involved; obviously the younger the child the greater is the growth loss. Arrest of one epiphysis in paired bones will lead to joint deformity. In the case illustrated, the radial epiphysis on the right has suffered complete growth arrest following a displaced lower radial epiphysis. The ulna has continued to grow at its usual rate; its distal end appears prominent on the dorsum of the wrist, and there is obvious deformity and impairment of function in the wrist. The normal left side is shown for comparison.

86. Fracture healing: As a result of the injury, (1) the periosteum may be completely or partly torn, (2) there is disruption of the Haversian systems with death of adjacent bone cells, (3) there may be tearing of muscle, especially on the convex side of the fracture, and damage to neighbouring nerves and blood vessels, (4) the skin may be broached in compound injuries, with risk of ingress of bacteria.

87. Fracture haematoma (a): Bleeding occurs from the bone ends, marrow vessels and damaged soft tissues, with the formation of a fracture haematoma which clots. (A closed fracture is illustrated.)

88. Fracture haematoma (b): The fracture haematoma is rapidly vascularised by the ingrowth of blood vessels from the surrounding tissues, and for some weeks there is rapid cellular activity. Fibrovascular tissue replaces the clot, collagen fibres are laid down and mineral salts are deposited.

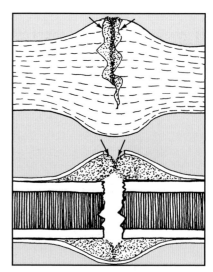

89. Subperiosteal bone: New woven bone is formed beneath the periosteum at the ends of the bone. The cells responsible are derived from the periosteum, which becomes stretched over these collars of new bone. If the blood supply is poor, or if it is disturbed by excessive mobility at the fracture site, cartilage may be formed instead and remain until a better blood supply is established.

90. Primary callus response: This remains active for *a few weeks only* (1). There is a much less vigorous formation of callus from the medullary cavity (2). Nevertheless, the capacity of the medulla to form new bone remains indefinitely throughout the healing of the fracture.

91. Bridging external callus (a): If the periosteum is incompletely torn, and there is no significant loss of bony apposition, the primary callus response may result in establishing external continuity of the fracture ('bridging external callus'). Cells lying in the outer layer of the periosteum itself proliferate to reconstitute the periosteum.

2

The diagnosis of fractures and principles of treatment

HOW TO DIAGNOSE A FRACTURE

1. HISTORY

In taking the history of a patient who may have a fracture, the following points may prove to be helpful, especially when there has been a traumatic incident.

1. What activity was being pursued at the time of the incident (e.g. taking part in a sport, driving a car, working at a height, etc.)?
2. What was the nature of the incident (e.g. a kick, a fall, a twisting injury, etc.)?
3. What was the magnitude of the applied forces? For example if a patient was injured in a fall, it is helpful to know how far he fell, if his fall was broken, the nature of the surface on which he landed, and how he landed; trivial violence may lead one to suspect a pathological fracture: severe violence makes the exclusion of multiple injuries particularly important.
4. What was the point of impact and the direction of the applied forces? In reducing a fracture, one of the principle methods employed is to reduplicate the causal forces in a reverse direction. If a fracture occurs close to the point of impact, additional remotely situated fractures must be excluded.
5. Is there any significance to be attached to the incident itself? For example, if there was a fall, was it precipitated by some underlying medical condition, such as a hypotensive attack, which requires separate investigation?
6. Where is the site of any pain, and what is its severity?
7. Is there loss of functional activity? For example, walking is seldom possible after any fracture of the femur or tibia; inability to weight bear after an accident is of great significance.
8. What is the patient's age? Note that while a young person may sustain bruising or a sprain following moderate trauma, an incident of comparative magnitude in an older patient may result in a fracture.

Diagnosis In some cases the diagnosis of fracture is unmistakable, e.g. when there is gross deformity of the central portion of a long bone or when the fracture is visible as in certain compound injuries. *In the majority of other cases, a fracture is suspected from the history and clinical examination, and confirmed by radiography of the region.*

2. Inspection (a): Begin by inspecting the limb most carefully, comparing one side with the other. Look for any *asymmetry of contour*, suggesting an underlying fracture which has displaced or angled.

3. Inspection (b): Look for any persisting *asymmetry of posture* of the limb, for example, persisting external rotation of the leg is a common feature in disimpacted fractures of the femoral neck.

4. Inspection (c): Look for local bruising of the skin suggesting a *point of impact* which may direct your attention locally or to a more distant level. For example, bruising over the knee from dashboard impact should direct your attention to the underlying patella, and also to the femoral shaft and hip.

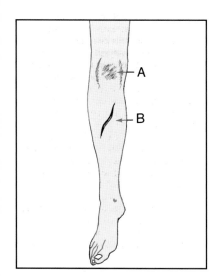

5. Inspection (d): Look for other tell-tale skin damage. For example (A) grazing, with or without ingraining of dirt in the wound, or friction burns, suggests an impact followed by rubbing of the skin against a resistant surface. (B) Lacerations suggest impact against a hard edge, tearing by a bone end, or splitting by compression against a hard surface.

6. Inspection (e): Note the presence of: (C) skin stretch marks, (D) band patterning of the skin, suggestive of both stretching and compression of the skin in a run-over injury, (E) pattern bruising, caused by severe compression which leads the skin to be imprinted with the weave marks of overlying clothing. Any of these abnormalities should lead you to suspect the integrity of the underlying bone.

7. Inspection (f): If the patient is seen shortly after the incident, note any localised swelling of the limb (1). Later, swelling tends to become more diffuse. Note the presence of any haematoma (2). A fracture may strip the skin from its local attachments (degloving injury); the skin comes to float on an underlying collection of blood which is continuous with the fracture haematoma.

8. Inspection (g): Note the colour of the injured limb, and compare it with the other. Slight cyanosis is suggestive of poor peripheral circulation; more marked cyanosis, venous obstruction; and whiteness, disturbance of the arterial supply. Feel the limb, and note the temperature at different levels, again comparing the sides. Check the pulses, and the rapidity of pinking-up after tissue compression.

9. Tenderness (a): Look for tenderness over the bone suspected of being fractured. Tenderness is invariably elicited over a fracture (1), but tenderness will also be found over any traumatised area, even though there is no underlying fracture (2). The important distinguishing feature is that in the case of a fracture tenderness will be elicited when the bone is palpated on any aspect (3).

10. Tenderness (b): In eliciting tenderness, once a tender area has been located the part should be palpated at the same level from another direction. For example, in many sprained wrists, tenderness will be elicited in the anatomical snuff-box – but not over the dorsal and palmar aspects of the scaphoid, which are tender if a fracture is present.

11. Palpation: The sharp edge of a fracture may be palpable. Note also the presence of localised oedema. This is a particularly useful sign over hair-line and stress fractures. The development of oedema may, however, take some hours to reach detectable proportions.

12. Other signs: If the fracture is mobile, moving the part may produce angulation or crepitus from the bone ends rubbing together. In addition, the patient will experience severe pain from such movement. These signs may be inadvertently observed during routine examination of the patient, but should not be sought unless the patient is unconscious and the diagnosis is in doubt.

13. Radiographic examination: In every case of suspected fracture, radiographic examination of the fracture is mandatory. Radiographs of the part will generally give a clear indication of the presence of a fracture and provide a sound basis for planning treatment. In the case where there is some clinical doubt, radiographs will reassure patient and surgeon and avert any later medicolegal criticism.

Radiographers in the United Kingdom receive thorough training in the techniques for the satisfactory visualisation of any suspect area, but it is essential that they in turn are given clear guidance as to the area under suspicion. The request form must be quite specific, otherwise mistakes may occur. At its simplest, the request must state *both the area to be visualised and the bone suspected of being fractured*. It is desirable to include the joints above and below the fracture. It need hardly be stressed that a thorough clinical examination should precede the completion of the radiographic request if repetition and the taking of unnecessary films are to be avoided.

The following table lists some of the commonest errors made in the filling in of request forms

Area suspected of fracture	Typical request	Error	Correct request
Scaphoid	X-ray wrist, ? fracture	Fractures of the scaphoid are difficult to visualise: a minimum of 3 specialised views is required. A fracture may not show on the standard wrist projections	X-ray scaphoid, ? fracture
Calcaneus	X-ray ankle, ? fracture X-ray foot, ? fracture	A tangential projection, with or without an additional oblique (along with the usual lateral), is necessary for satisfactory visualisation of the calcaneus. These views are not taken routinely when an X-ray examination of the foot or ankle is called for	X-ray calcaneus, ? fracture
Neck of femur	'X-ray femur, ? fracture'	Poor centring of the radiographs may render the fracture invisible	'X-ray hip, ? fracture neck of femur' or 'X-ray to exclude fracture of femoral neck'
Tibial plateau or tibial spines	'X-ray tibia, ? fracture'	Poor centring may render the fracture invisible, or the area may not be included on the film	'X-ray upper third tibia to exclude fracture of tibial plateau'

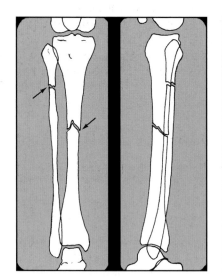

14. The standard projections: These are an *anteroposterior (AP) and lateral.* Ideally the beam should be centred over the area of suspected fracture, with visualisation of the proximal *and* distal joints. This is especially important in the paired long bones where, for example, a fracture of the tibia at one level may be accompanied by a fibular fracture at another.

15. Comparison films: Where there is some difficulty in interpreting the radiographs (e.g. in the elbow region in children where the epiphyseal structures are continually changing, or where there is some unexplained shadow, or a congenital abnormality) films of the other side should be taken for direct comparison.

16. Oblique projections: In the case of the hand and foot, an oblique projection may be helpful when the lateral gives rise to confusion due to the superimposition of many structures. Such oblique projections may have to be specifically requested when they are not part of an X-ray department's routine.

in the case of hepatitis C (circa 1 in 5000). Septic reactions are rare, but commoner with platelet concentrates which are stored at room temperature.

6. Reactions. Acute haemolytic reactions from mismatched blood require immediate cessation of blood administration and a full investigation which should include a haematocrit to check for the presence of haemolysis, culture of the patient's and donor's blood to exclude bacterial contamination, repeat cross-matching, a full blood count and examination of red cell morphology, and a Coomb's test. The donor blood should be returned to the blood bank and advice sought from the haematologist regarding any further investigation thought desirable. All aspects should be rigorously documented. The urinary output must be carefully monitored while an attempt is made to obtain a brisk diuresis. Severe reactions can occur from 30 mL of mismatched blood, are life threatening, and may require dialysis.

Non-haemolytic reactions, often with severe associated urticaria, usually occur after administration of larger quantities of whole blood or packed cells, and may often be controlled with intravenous benadryl. Washed red cells may be given if further transfusion is required.

PERSISTING CIRCULATORY INSTABILITY

Where rapid, appropriate transfusion fails to control the situation, the commonest cause is continued bleeding. In most cases the site is obvious.

1. External haemorrhage accompanying limb injuries should be readily controlled if this has not already been done.

2. Continuing blood loss from intrathoracic injuries should be obvious. Assuming that a haemothorax has been diagnosed and treated by the insertion of a chest drain, the quantity and rate of loss may be evaluated by monitoring the volumes in the collection bottle(s). This may be used to assess the need for exploration to control persisting haemorrhage.

3. Massive bleeding from within the abdominal cavity usually requires immediate laparotomy, but it is essential to be sure that the bleeding is not from the pelvis. (An unstable fracture of the pelvis and a negative abdominal ultrasound would be a contraindication for laparotomy.)

The commonest causes of intra-abdominal haemorrhage are tearing of the liver, spleen or mesentery, and all are potentially amenable to surgery.

4. Haemorrhage accompanying fractures of the pelvis. This is most common in unstable fractures involving the sacroiliac joints; the bleeding may be from the pelvic plexus of veins or from damage to the iliac arteries. In the first instance, especially if there is little sacroiliac disruption, an external pelvic fixator should be employed, and replacement efforts renewed. If the sacroiliac joint is disrupted and the situation fails to resolve, a (posterior) C-clamp should be applied. If circulatory instability persists, then exploration may be needed as a last resort. Diffuse bleeding from the pelvic venous plexus is generally best controlled by packing. On rare occasions selective embolisation or ligature of the iliac arteries may be necessary.

5. Haemorrhage from the urinary tract is seldom very severe, but nevertheless may be a problem. It should be suspected if there is a haematuria or some other indication (such as the presence of a fracture of the pelvis of appropriate pattern). The diagnosis may be clarified by an intravenous pyelogram, a cystogram, or a urethrogram.

PRIORITIES OF TREATMENT

The presence of other matters of importance may well have been noted in the initial survey, but their management may have to be deferred until resuscitation is under way. Note the following:

Head injury

1. Where there is a head injury the following procedures should be followed:

(a) The unconscious patient should be intubated to minimise the risks of cerebral hypoxia.

(b) A complete neurological examination must be carried out and the results charted, using a suitable set of protocols (such as the Glasgow Coma Scale, see below); the examination should be repeated at regular intervals. Of particular significance is (i) a history of a post-traumatic lucid interval; (ii) a history of progressive deterioration in the level of consciousness; (iii) focal neurological signs; (iv) a rising blood pressure and falling pulse rate.

Glasgow Coma Scale

A patient is defined as being comatose if he does not open his eyes, if he does not obey commands, and if he does not utter recognisable words. The severity of the coma may be assessed by assigning a value to the eye, motor and verbal responses, and summing these. By repeating the examinations at regular intervals progress may be monitored, and any deterioration (suggesting intracranial complications) recognised at an early stage.

Variable	Score
Eye-opening (E)	
Spontaneous	4
To speech	3
To pain	2
Nil	1
Best motor response (M)	
Obeys	6
Localises	5
Withdraws	4
Abnormal flexion	3
Extensor response	2
Nil	1
Verbal response	
Oriented	5
Confused conversation	4
Inappropriate words	3
Incomprehensible sounds	2
Nil	1

The coma score = E+M+V, with a value of 3 being the worst possible response, and 15 the best. A value of less than 7 indicates severe coma, 8–12 moderate, and 13–14 mild. Severe injuries are infrequent, and most patients who develop haematomas requiring surgery are classified as moderate or minor on admission.

(c) Where there is evidence of increased intracranial pressure further investigation with a CT scan should be carried out. If an extradural haematoma is discovered its immediate evacuation should be undertaken. If a subdural haematoma is found this should be also promptly removed. If there is evidence of diffuse cerebral oedema, surgery is contraindicated, and an infusion of a hyperosmolar solution of Mannitol may be commenced. Where appropriate, monitoring of the intracranial pressure may be carried out using a catheter inserted into the lateral ventricle.

As far as the treatment of fractures accompanying a head injury is concerned, the following points should be noted. Where the head injury requires urgent investigative procedures or operative intervention (for example an extradural haemorrhage with deterioration in the level of consciousness) this will take priority over the local treatment of most fractures. A combined procedure may often be planned with advantage but certainly in all cases some estimate should be made as to when definitive treatment of the fracture is likely to be possible. Depending on that interval there is the choice of a variety of initial procedures which may include the application of sterile dressings or light packing of open wounds, supporting an injured limb with sandbags or an inflatable splint in such a position that the distal circulation is maintained, or the use of light temporary plaster splintage.

2. Where there is a head injury in which the immediate prognosis is hopeless any temporary splintage of the fracture should be retained but no fresh treatment planned.
3. Where no active neurosurgical treatment is contemplated and the prognosis regarded as very poor but not absolutely hopeless, it is usually possible to devise some simple measures to give reasonable support to the injured part but at the same time permitting more definitive treatment in the near future should unexpected improvement occur.

Cardiac tamponade: intrathoracic rupture of the aorta Prompt drainage of an intrapericardial haematoma may be a life-saving measure and aortic rupture may not be immediately fatal. Widening and squaring-off of the mediastinal shadow on the chest radiographs, and cardiac distress should alert suspicion of these injuries. Further investigation may be required by echocardiography, angiography or CT scan. Thoracotomy may be required (with by-pass facilities in the case of intrathoracic rupture of the aorta). Thoracotomy may also be indicated where there is a tracheal, bronchial or oesophageal injury, or a penetrating injury to the mediastinum.

Visceral complications Most require exploration and surgical correction. Injury to the liver, spleen and kidneys may give rise to severe intra-abdominal haemorrhage. Haemorrhage may also follow mesenteric tears and ruptures of the stomach and intestine with which the problems of perforation are also associated. Intra-abdominal haemorrhage is best diagnosed by ultrasound. Perforation may be suspected in the absence of bowel sounds and where there is loss of liver dullness. Plain lateral recumbent abdominal radiographs may be of some help, but peritoneal lavage is often invaluable: the presence of bile or digestive contents may be diagnostic. CT scans are sometimes helpful, especially in diagnosing injuries to the pancreas. Rupture of the diaphragm is often missed in cases of blunt abdominal trauma. Its presence may be concealed if there is an accompanying chest injury. Diagnosis may require chest films taken while a contrast medium is administered by nasogastric tube. In the case of the urinary tract, examination of the urine for blood; an intravenous pyelogram and cystogram, and in certain pelvic fractures a urethrogram may also be employed (see Complications of Pelvic Fractures).

Eye and facio-maxillary injuries Perforating injuries of the eye and major facial injuries require immediate surgery at the beginning of the primary period. Minor facial soft tissue injuries and fractures may be delayed till later during the primary period. Unstable facial fractures are generally stabilised during the primary period, with major reconstructive procedures being delayed until facial swelling has subsided.

Spinal fractures Where there is an unstable fracture with no neurological involvement, or incomplete neurological involvement, stabilisation of the fracture is essential during the primary period to prevent deterioration. Where there is evidence of progressive neurological involvement (e.g. from compression of the cord by bone or disc fragments), surgery is also indicated in the primary phase. (See under spine p. 251.)

Vascular injuries In the presence of continuing blood loss or ischaemia, further investigation may be required prior to exploration if the nature and extent of any injury is not apparent. (See p. 104.)

EVALUATION OF PATIENTS WITH MULTIPLE INJURIES

Trauma scoring; hospital trauma index; injury severity score; damage control orthopaedics Several systems have been developed in an attempt to assess the severity of injuries. These may be used as an alert for the need for prompt and expert treatment; they may give an indication of the prognosis; and over a period they may be used statistically to evaluate the performance of a team, unit or hospital, or to draw attention to some injury pattern where treatment efforts might be profitably concentrated.

The two main systems in use are the Abbreviated Injury Scale (AIS), and the Hospital Trauma Index (HTI). Both classifications are largely comparable, and for normal working purposes grade injuries into five degrees of severity:

0 = None
1 = Minor
2 = Moderate
3 = Major, but not life-threatening
4 = Severe, life-threatening, but survival probable
5 = Critical, survival uncertain.

Where the injury is isolated (i.e. the case is not one of multiple injuries), there is no problem and the grade into which the injury falls is used as required.

Where there are multiple injuries the addition of the values obtained from the AIS or HTI tables does not give an accurate indication of severity, being overly pessimistic regarding outcome. It has been found, however, that if the grade figures are manipulated, a figure is reached which can be used with some measure of accuracy as a prognostic indicator in cases of multiple injury.

In practice, the patient's three worst injuries are assessed and the relevant grade numbers are each squared before being added together. If several injuries lie within the same area, only the worst is selected. The break point for the resultant sum is in the area of 50. The following points may be noted:

- Score < 10: death rare in any patient under the age of 50 years.
- Score 10–20: mortality 4–30%, depending on age.
- Score > 50: only rare survival, and only in exceptional circumstances and with prompt treatment by specialised staff. In this group nearly all the deaths occur within the first week, and half within the first hour.

In all groups the mortality rate rises with age; for example when the score lies between 10 and 19, the mortality rate in the 70+ year age group is more than 8 times the rate for those under 50 years. The effects of age are somewhat paradoxically most noticeable when the injury severity scores are comparatively low.

- Score 10–15: the response to treatment of cases within this band does most to throw light on the evaluation of the standard of medical care offered by any team or department. Cases within this group are sufficiently ill to be adversely affected by poor care; but they are not so ill that no matter how expert the treatment they cannot survive.

Summary of hospital trauma index: Six areas must be considered when using this method of assessment: respiratory, cardiovascular, nervous system, abdominal, extremities, skin and subcutaneous. A seventh area of complications can be included for assessments, which are made at a late stage.

Respiratory

1	(minor)	Chest discomfort – minimal findings
2	(moderate)	Simple rib or sternal fracture, chest wall contusion with pleuritic pain
3	(major)	Multiple rib or first rib fracture, haemothorax, pneumothorax
4	(severe)	Open chest wound, flail chest, tension pneumothorax with normal BP, simple laceration of diaphragm
5	(critical)	Acute cyanotic respiratory failure, aspiration, tension pneumothorax with lowered BP, complicated laceration of diaphragm

Cardiovascular

1	(minor)	Less than 500 mL blood loss (less than 10% blood volume) with no change in perfusion
2	(moderate)	Blood loss of 500–1000 mL (10–20% blood volume), decreased skin perfusion but normal urinary output, myocardial contusion with normal BP
3	(major)	Blood loss of 1000–1500 mL (20–30% blood volume), decreased skin perfusion, slight decrease in urinary output, tamponade, BP 80 mmHg
4	(severe)	Blood loss 1500–2000 ml (30–40% blood volume), decreased skin perfusion, urinary output less than 10 mL per hour, tamponade, conscious, BP less than 80 mmHg
5	(critical)	Blood loss in excess of 2000 mL (40–50% loss of blood volume), restless, coma, cardiac contusion or arrythmia, BP unrecordable. (Note that the previously described classification of haemorrhage into four grades has been slightly altered for this 5 point scoring system.)

Nervous system

1	(minor)	Head injury with or without scalp laceration, but no loss of consciousness or skull fracture
2	(moderate)	Head injury with unconsciousness of under 15 minutes, skull fracture, cervical pain with minimal findings, one facial fracture
3	(major)	Head injury with coma of more than 15 minutes, depressed skull fracture, cervical spine fracture or dislocation with positive neurological findings, multiple facial fractures
4	(severe)	Head injury with coma in excess of 1 hour or with positive neurological findings, cervical spine fracture or dislocation with paraplegia
5	(critical)	Head injury with coma and no response to stimuli up to 24 hours, cervical spine fracture or dislocation with quadriplegia

Abdominal

1	(minor)	Mild abdominal wall, flank or back pain with tenderness but no peritoneal signs
2	(moderate)	Acute flank, back or abdominal discomfort and tenderness, fracture of a seventh to twelfth rib
3	(major)	Isolated injury to liver (minor), small bowel, spleen, kidney, body of pancreas, mesentery, ureter, urethra, fractures of ribs 7–12
4	(severe)	Two major injuries: of rupture of the liver, bladder, head of pancreas, duodenum, colon, (large) of mesentery
5	(critical)	Two severe injuries: crushing of liver; major vascular, including thoracic or abdominal aorta, vena cava, iliacs, hepatic veins

Extremities

1	(minor)	Minor sprain or fracture not involving a long bone
2	(moderate)	Closed fracture of humerus, clavicle, radius, ulna, tibia, fibula, involvement of a single nerve
3	(major)	Multiple moderate fractures, open moderate, closed femur, stable pelvis, major dislocation, major nerve injury
4	(severe)	Two major long bone fractures, open fracture of femur, crushing or amputation of limb, unstable pelvic fracture
5	(critical)	Two severe or multiple major fractures

Skin and subcutaneous

1	(minor)	Less than 5% burns, abrasions, contusions, lacerations
2	(moderate)	Burns of 5–15%, extensive contusions, avulsions 8–15 cm, lacerations totalling 30 cm in length
3	(major)	Burns of 15–30%, avulsions of 30 cm
4	(severe)	Burns of 30–45%, avulsion of leg or arm
5	(critical)	Burn of 45–60%

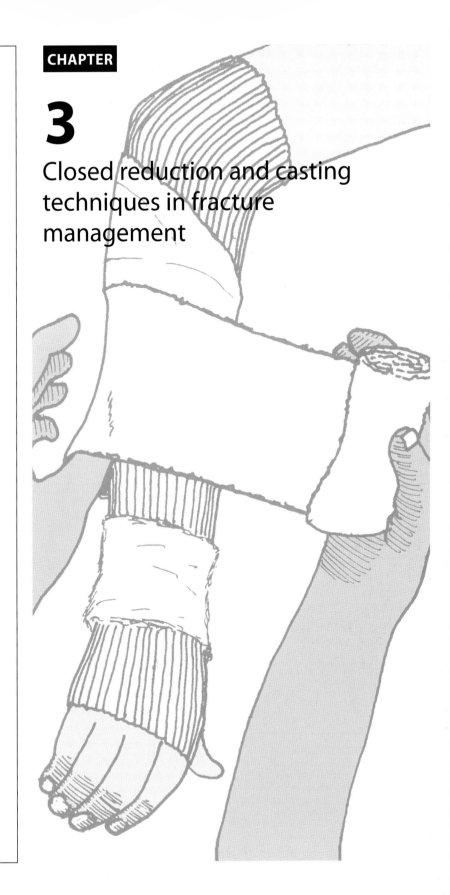

3

Closed reduction and casting techniques in fracture management

1. Closed reduction of fractures: Basic techniques (a): The direction and magnitude of the causal force (1) and the deformity (2) are related, and may be worked out from the history, the appearance of the limb and the radiographs. Any force required to correct the displacement of a fracture is applied in the opposite direction (3).

2. Basic techniques (b): The first step in most closed reductions is to apply traction – generally in the line of the limb (1). Traction will lead to the disimpaction of most fractures (2) and this may occur almost immediately in the relaxed patient under general anaesthesia. Traction will also lead to reduction of shortening (3), and in most cases to reduction of the deformity (4).

3. Basic techniques (c): Any residual angulation following the application of traction may be corrected by using the heel of the hand under the fracture (1) and applying pressure distally with the other (2).

6. Basic techniques (f): After reduction of the fracture it must be prevented from redisplacing until it has united. The methods include the following:
Plaster fixation (p. 57).
Skin and skeletal traction (for examples, see p. 328).
Thomas splint (see p. 329).
Cast bracing (see p. 334).
External fixation (see p. 79).
For common methods of internal fixation see Chapter 4.

4. Basic techniques (d): In some fractures there may be difficulty in reduction due to prominent bony spikes or soft tissue interposition. Reduction may sometimes be achieved by initially increasing the angulation prior to manipulation. This method of unlocking the fragments must be pursued with care to avoid damage to surrounding vessels and nerves.

5. Basic techniques (e): The effectiveness of reduction may be assessed by noting the appearance of the limb (1), by palpation, especially in long bone fractures (2), by absence of telescoping (i.e. axial compression along the line of the limb does not lead to further shortening) (3), and by check radiographs.

7. Protection of the skin: Stockingette:
A layer of stockingette is usually applied next to the skin (1). This has several functions: it helps prevent the limb hairs becoming caught in the plaster, it facilitates the conduction of perspiration from the limb, it removes any roughness caused by the ends of the plaster and it may aid in the subsequent removal of the plaster. After the plaster has been applied, the stockingette is turned back (2).

8. Stockingette *ctd*: After the stockingette has been reflected, excess is removed, leaving 3–4 cm only at each end (3). The loose edge of the stockingette is then secured with a turn or two of a plaster bandage (if a complete plaster is being applied) or with the encircling gauze bandage in the case of a slab.

9. Wool roll: A layer of wool should be used to protect bony prominences (e.g. the distal ulna). In complete plasters, where swelling is anticipated, several layers of wool may be applied over the length of the limb; the initial layer of stockingette may be omitted. A layer of wool may also be substituted for stockingette under a slab, and indeed many like to use a layer of wool under any type of cast. Wool roll is also advisable where an electric saw is used for plaster removal.

10. Felt: Where friction is likely to occur over bony prominences, protection may be given with felt strips or felt cut-outs, fashioned to isolate the area to be relieved (e.g. the vertebral and iliac spines, the pubis and manubrium in plaster jackets). Adhesive felt should not be applied directly to the skin if skin eruptions are to be avoided.

11. Plaster slabs (a): These consist of several layers of plaster bandage and may be used for the treatment of minor injuries or where potentially serious swelling may be anticipated in a fracture. In their application, slabs are cut to length (1), and trimmed as required (2) to fit the limb before being applied (3). Slabs may also be used as foundations or reinforcements of complete plasters.

12. Plaster slabs (b): If a slab dispenser is available, measure the length of slab required and cut to length. A single slab of six layers of bandage will usually suffice for a child. In a large adult, two slab thicknesses may be necessary. In a small adult, one slab thickness may be adequate with local reinforcement.

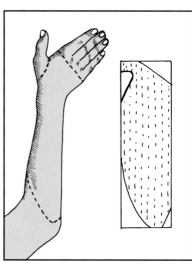

13. Plaster slabs (c): Alternatively, manufacture a slab by repeated folding of a plaster bandage, using say 8–10 thicknesses in an adult and six in a child as described (1). Turn in the end of the bandage (2) so that when the slab is dipped the upper layer does not fall out of alignment.

14. Plaster slabs (d): Ideally the slab should be trimmed with plaster scissors so that it will fit the limb without being folded over. For example, a slab for an undisplaced greenstick fracture of the distal radius should stretch from the metacarpal heads to the olecranon. It may be measured (1) and trimmed as shown, with a tongue (2) to lie between the thumb and index.

15. Plaster slabs (e): In a Colles fracture (see p. 196) where the hand should be placed in a position of ulnar deviation, the slab should be trimmed to accommodate this position, a stage that is often omitted in error. The preceding two plaster slabs are examples of dorsal slabs.

16. Plaster slabs (f): An anterior slab may be used as a foundation for a scaphoid plaster (see p. 209), or to treat an injury in which the wrist is held in dorsiflexion (measuring from a point just distal to the elbow crease with the elbow at 90°, to the proximal skin crease in the palm). The proximal end is rounded (1) while the distal lateral corner is trimmed for the thenar mass (2).

17. Plaster slabs (g): For the ankle (1) a plain untrimmed slab may be used, measuring from the metatarsal heads to the upper calf, 3–4 cm distal to a point behind the tibial tubercle. For the foot (2) where the toes require support, choose the tips of the toes as the distal point.

18. Plaster slabs (h): Owing to the abrupt change in direction of the slab at the ankle, the slab requires cutting on both sides so that it may be smoothed down with local overlapping. A back slab may be further strengthened by a long U-slab with its limbs lying medially and laterally.

19. Plaster slabs (i): The same technique of side cutting is required for long arm plaster slabs (1). These are measured as indicated from the upper arm to the metacarpal heads, with a cut-out at the thumb as in a Colles plaster slab (2).

20. Plaster slabs (j): Wetting the slab: hold it carefully at both ends, immerse completely in tepid water, lift out and momentarily bunch up at an angle to expel excess water. Plaster-setting time is decreased by both hot and soft water.

21. Plaster slabs (k): Now consolidate the layers of the slab. If a plaster table is available, quickly place the slab on the surface and, with one movement with the heels of the hands, press the layers firmly together. (Retained air reduces the ultimate strength of the plaster and leads to cracking or separation of the layers.)

22. Plaster slabs (l): Alternatively, consolidate the layers by holding the plaster at one end and pulling between two adducted fingers (1). Repeat the procedure from the other edge (2).

23. Plaster slabs (m): Carefully position the slab on the limb and smooth out with the hands so that the slab fits closely to the contours of the limb without rucking or the formation of sore-making ridges on its inferior surface.

24. Plaster slabs (n): At this stage any weak spots should be reinforced. Where there is a right-angled bend in a plaster – for example at the elbow or the ankle – two small slabs made from 10 cm (4″) plaster bandages may be used as triangular reinforcements at either site. A similar small slab may be used to reinforce the back of the wrist.

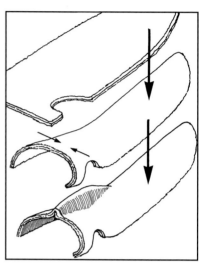

25. Plaster slabs (o): In the case of a long-leg plaster slab, additional strengthening at the thigh and knee is always necessary, and this may be achieved by the use of two additional (15 cm) (6″) slabs.

26. Plaster slabs (p): Where even greater strength is required, the plaster may be girdered. For example, for the wrist, make a small slab of six thicknesses of 10 cm (4″) bandage and pinch up in the centre (1). Dip the reinforcement, apply, and smooth down to form a T-girder over the dorsum (2).

27. Plaster slabs (q): Girdering may also be achieved without a separate onlay.
The basic plaster slab is pinched up locally after being applied to the limb. Care must be taken to avoid undue ridging of the interior surface.

30. Complete POP technique: 1. The skin should be protected as previously described, using where applicable stockingette, wool roll and felt. 2. The following sizes of plaster bandage are recommended for normal application:

Upper arm and forearm	15 cm (6″)
Wrist	10 cm (4″)
Thumb and fingers	7.5 cm (3″)
Trunk and hip	20 cm (8″)
Thigh and leg	20 cm (8″)
Ankle and foot	15 cm (6″)

28. Bandaging (a): Bandages used to secure plaster slabs should be of open weave (cotton or muslin) and be thoroughly wetted. This is to avoid tightening from shrinkage after coming in contact with the slab. Secure the end of the bandage between the thumb and fingers, and squeeze several times under water.

29. Bandaging (b): Apply to the limb firmly, but without too much pressure (1).
Do not use reverse turns, which tend to produce local constrictions. The ends of the underlying stockingette may be turned back and secured with the last few turns of the bandage (2). On completion, secure the bandage with a small piece of wetted plaster bandage.

31. Plaster bandage wetting (a): Plaster bandages should be dipped in tepid water. Secure the end of the bandage with one hand to prevent the end becoming lost in the mass of wet bandage. Hold the bandage lightly with the other hand without compression. Immerse at an angle of 45°, and keep under water until bubbles stop rising.

32. Plaster bandage wetting (b): Remove excess water by gently compressing in an axial direction and twisting slightly. Alternatively, pull the bandage through the encircled thumb and index while lightly gripping the bandage.

33. Plaster bandage application (a): Most moulding of the plaster will be required at the wrist in upper limb plasters, and at the ankle in lower limb plasters. It is often useful to apply the more proximal parts first, so that moulding can be more profitably carried out against a set or nearly set cuff of plaster on the forearm or calf (i.e. start a forearm plaster at the elbow, and a below-knee plaster at the tibial tubercle).

34. Plaster bandage application (b): Roll each bandage without stretching if there is no wool beneath; if there is a layer of wool, and no swelling is anticipated, a little even pressure may be applied to compress the wool to half thickness. Plain tucks may be used distally to ensure a smooth fit, but figure-of-eight or reverse turns should not be used if local constriction is to be avoided.

35. Plaster bandage application (c): After the application of each bandage smooth the layers down to exclude any trapped air and consolidate the plaster. A second and if necessary a third bandage may be applied to complete the proximal portion. Each bandage should extend 2–3 cm distal to the previous, and be well smoothed down. The distal part may then be completed, and the hand or foot portion moulded before setting is complete.

36. Plaster bandage application (d): Where possible the assistant should hold the limb in such a way that the surgeon has a clear run while applying the plaster (1). Where support must be given to a part included in the plaster, the flats of the hands should be used, and the hands eased proximally and distally to avoid local indentation. Where slabs are used, try to let gravity assist rather than hinder (2).

37. Removal of rings (a): Wherever possible rings should be removed in case finger swelling leads to distal gangrene.
A tight ring can generally be coaxed from a finger if it is well coated with olive oil or a similar lubricant. If this fails, the finger may sometimes be sufficiently compressed by binding it with, for example, macramé twine to allow removal as shown.

38. Removal of rings (b): Otherwise a ring may be cut with a ring cutter (1) or a saw cut may be made with a fine tooth hack-saw on to a spatula (2) to spring the ring. Ring removal is nevertheless sometimes obsessively pursued. If significant swelling is unlikely, the ring loose below the knuckle, the patient intelligent and the potential danger is indicated, it may be retained with acceptable safety.

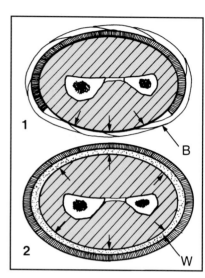

39. Plaster precautions (a): After an acute injury, if much swelling is anticipated (1) use a plaster slab in preference to a complete plaster. The retaining bandages have more 'give' than plaster, and are more readily cut in an emergency. (2) If a slab does not give sufficient support, then allow for swelling with a generous layer of wool beneath the plaster. (W=wool; B= bandage.)

40. Plaster precautions (b): Consider splitting any complete plaster. This should be done *routinely* after any operative procedure when swelling may be considerable (from tourniquet release, postoperative oedema, etc.). Use a sharp knife and cut down through the plaster to the underlying wool. (The wool protects the skin.) This should be done immediately after application of the plaster before it has had time to dry out.

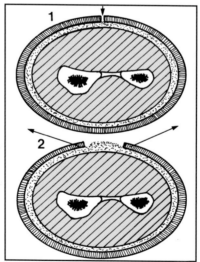

41. Plaster precautions (c): Be sure the plaster has been *completely* divided down to the wool along its whole length (1). (Any remaining strands will act dangerously as constricting bands.) You should be able to see the wool quite clearly. The plaster edges should spring apart by 5–10 mm or they may be eased apart by the handle of the knife, thereby dynamically relieving any underlying pressure (2).

42. Elevation (a): Wherever possible, the injured limb should be elevated. In the case of the hand and forearm in a patient who has been admitted, the limb may be secured in stockingette (or in a roller towel using safety pins) attached to a drip stand at the side of the bed. Elevation should be maintained at least until swelling is beginning to resolve.

43. Elevation (b): In the case of the ambulant patient a sling may be used, provided the arm is kept high enough (1).
If the sling is too slack the arm will hang down, encouraging oedema (2).

44. Elevation (c): In the case of the lower limb, the leg may be elevated on pillows (1). The end of the bed may be raised on an A-frame or on chairs (2). The ambulant patient should be advised to keep the foot as high as possible on a couch or chair whenever he is at rest.

45. Exercise: Those parts free of plaster should be exercised as frequently as possible: for example, the fingers in a Colles fracture (and later the elbow and shoulder). The patient should be shown how she should curl the fingers into full flexion and then fully extend them. She should be given clear instructions as to how frequently she should perform these exercises (e.g. for 5 minutes every waking hour).

Instructions for Patients in Plaster of Paris Splints

A. (1) If fingers or toes become swollen blue, painful or stiff, raise limb.

    (2) If no improvement in half an hour call in Doctor or return to hospital immediately.

B. (1) Exercise all joints not included in plaster—especially fingers and toes

    (2) If you have been fitted with a walking plaster walk in it.

    (3) If plaster becomes loose or cracked—report to hospital as soon as possible.

46. The patient who is being allowed home must be given clear warnings to return should the circulation appear in any way to be impaired. Inform the patient or, where appropriate, a relative who will be looking after the patient. It is also useful to reinforce this by pasting an instruction label (such as the one illustrated) directly to the plaster.

47. Aftercare of patients in plaster: Note the following: (a): *Is there swelling?* Swelling of the fingers or toes is common in patients being treated in plaster, but the patient must be examined carefully for other signs which might suggest that circulatory impairment is the cause, rather than the local response to trauma. If there is no evidence of circulatory impairment, the limb should be elevated and movements encouraged.

48. (b): *Is there discolouration of the toes or fingers?* Compare one side with the other; bluish discolouration, especially in conjunction with oedematous swelling distally, suggests that swelling of the limb within the plaster has reached such a level as to impair the venous return, and appropriate action must be taken.

49. (c): *Is there any evidence of arterial obstruction?* Note the five Ps: intense pain, paralysis of finger or toe flexors, paraesthesiae in fingers or toes, pallor of the skin with disturbed capillary return, and 'perishing cold' feel of the fingers and toes. Arterial obstruction requires *immediate*, positive action. (Clinical findings of a similar nature, along with pain on passive movements of the fingers or toes is found in the compartment syndromes: see p. 105).

50. Treatment of suspected circulatory impairment (1): (i) Elevate the limb (ii) In the case of a plaster slab, cut through the encircling bandages and underlying wool (2) until the *skin is fully exposed*, and ease back the edges of the plaster shell until it is apparent that it is not constricting the limb in any way.

51. Treatment (2): Where the plaster is a complete one, split the plaster throughout its entire length. *Ease* back the edges of the cast to free the limb on each side of the midline. *Divide* all the overlying wool and stockingette and turn it back till skin is exposed. The same applies to any dressing swabs hardened with blood clot.

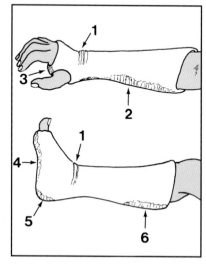

52. Treatment (3): If the circulation has been restored, gently pack wool between the cut edges of the plaster (1) and firmly apply an encircling crepe bandage (2). If this is not done, there is risk of extensive skin ('plaster') blistering locally. If the circulation is not restored, re-appraise the position of the fracture and suspect major vessel involvement. *On no account adopt an expectant and procrastinating policy.*

53. (d): *Can the plaster be completed?* If the plaster consists of a back-slab or shell, completion depends on your assessment of the present swelling, and your prediction of any further swelling. Most plasters may be completed after 48 hours; but if swelling is very marked completion should be delayed for a further 2 days, or until it is showing signs of subsiding.

54. (e): *Is the plaster intact?* Look for evidence of cracking, especially in the region of the joints (1). In arm plasters, look for anterior softening (2) and softening in the palm (3). In the leg, look for softening of the sole piece (4), the heel (5) and calf (6). Any weak areas should be reinforced by the application of more plaster locally.

55. (f): *Is the plaster causing restriction of movement?* Look especially for encroachment of the palm piece on the ulnar side of the hand, restricting MP joint flexion (1). In forearm plasters, look also for restriction of elbow movements. In below-knee plasters, note if the plaster is digging in when the knee is flexed (2). Trim the plaster as appropriate (3).

56. (g): *Is the plaster too short?* Note especially the Colles-type plaster with inadequate grip of the forearm (1); note the below-knee plaster which does not reach the tibial tuberosity (2) and which, apart from affording unsatisfactory support of an ankle fracture, will inevitably cause friction against the shin. Extend the defective plasters where appropriate (3).

57. (h): *Has the plaster become too loose?* A plaster may become loose as a result of the subsidence of limb swelling and from muscle wasting. If a plaster is slack, then the support afforded to the underlying fracture may become inadequate. Assess looseness by attempting to move the plaster proximally and distally, while noting its excursion in each direction.

58. *Has the plaster become too loose? Ctd:* In the leg, grasp the plaster and pull it distally; note how far the toes disappear into the plaster. If a plaster is loose, it should be changed unless (i) union is nearing completion and risks of slipping are minimal or (ii) a good position is held and the risks of slipping while the plaster is being changed are thought to be greater than the risks of slipping in a loose plaster.

59. (i): *Is the patient complaining of localised pain?* Localised pain, especially over a bony prominence, may indicate inadequate local padding, local pressure and pressure sore formation. In a child it may sometimes suggest a foreign body pushed in under the plaster. In all cases, the affected area should be inspected by cutting a window in the plaster and replacing it after examination.

60. How to remove a plaster: plaster slabs: Plaster shells or slabs are easily removed by cutting the encircling open weave bandages which hold them in position. Care must be taken to avoid nicking the skin, and Bohler scissors are helpful in this respect.

61. Removing complete plasters: Using shears (a): The heel of the shears must lie between the plaster and the limb. Subcutaneous bony prominences such as the shaft of the ulna (1) should be avoided to lessen the risks of skin damage and pain. Instead, the route of the shears should be planned to lie over compressible soft-tissue masses (2).

62. Using shears (b): If possible, avoid cutting over a concavity. If the wrist is in moderate palmar flexion as in a Colles plaster, the plaster should be removed by a dorsal cut (1). In a scaphoid plaster, the dorsal route should be avoided (2) and the plaster removed anteriorly.

63. Using shears (c): Where there is the right-angled bend of the ankle to negotiate, it is often helpful to make two vertical cuts down through the sole piece (1) and turn it down (2). This then gives access for the shears to make a vertical cut behind the lateral malleolus (3) and then skirt forwards over the peronei (4). The remaining plaster may then be sprung open.

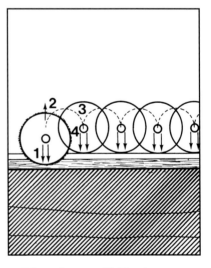

64. Using shears (d): Keep the lower handle (L) parallel to the plaster, or even a little depressed. Lift up the upper handle (U); push the shears forward with the lower handle so that the plaster fills the throat of the shears. Maintaining a slight pushing force, all the cutting action may be performed with the upper handle, moving it up and down like a beer pump.

65. Using a plaster saw (a): Plaster saws may be used for removing or cutting windows in plasters, but they should be used with caution and treated with respect. Do not use a plaster saw unless there is a layer of wool between the plaster and the skin. Do not use it over bony prominences and do not use if the blade is bent, broken or blunt. *Note:* the blade does not rotate but oscillates.

66. Using a plaster saw (b): Electric saws are noisy, and the apprehensive patient should be reassured. Cut down through the plaster at one level (1); the note will change as soon as it is through; remove the saw (2) and shift it laterally about an inch (2.5 cm) (3) and repeat (4). *Do not* slide the saw laterally in shallow cuts; the cutting movement should be up and down.

67. Polymer resin casts: Most use bandages of cotton (e.g. Bayer's Baycast®), fibreglass (Smith & Nephew's Dynacast XR®) or polypropylene (3M's Primacast®), impregnated with a resin which hardens on contact with water. Advantages include: (1) strength combined with lightness, (2) rapid setting (5–10 min) and curing, reaching maximum strength in 30 min (cf. plasters whose slow 'drying out' period of about 48 hours may lead if unprotected to cracking), (3) water resistance combined with porosity (although wetting of the inner layers should still be avoided), (4) radiolucence.

Disadvantages include: (1) high item cost – but their durability reduces demands on staff and transport, (2) they generally mould less well than plaster, and are more unyielding.

After acute injuries, where further swelling is likely, plaster is generally the more suitable casting material; it can be carefully moulded to the part giving particularly good support, and where necessary it can be applied in the form of a slab. When swelling subsides, and the stability of the fracture is not in doubt, a resin cast may be substituted. Where little swelling is anticipated in a stable fresh fracture, a resin cast may be used from the outset. Where a cast is likely to be abused (e.g. in wet weather where an extroverted teenager requires support for an ankle injury) there is much to be said for using a resin cast, and of course it is possible to reinforce an ordinary plaster cast with an outer resin bandage.

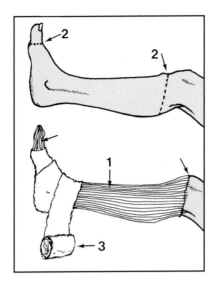

68. Application (a): Apply conforming stockingette (1) to the limb: ensure that it extends 3–5 cm (1–2″) beyond the proposed limits of the cast itself (2). Next, apply a layer of padding (3), paying particular care to protect the bony prominences. Where it is necessary to resist exposure to water or to moisture, a synthetic water-resistant orthopaedic padding may be used (e.g. Smith & Nephew's Soffban®).

69. Application (b): Open each bandage pack only as required to avoid premature curing. Wear gloves to prevent the resin adhering to your skin or causing sensitisation. Immerse the bandage in warm water for 2–5 seconds, squeezing it two to four times to accelerate setting. Fewer bandages will be required than with plaster, e.g. a below-knee cast in an adult may be applied with two 7.5 cm (3″) and one to two 10 cm (4″) bandages. Use the smaller sizes for the areas requiring a high degree of conformity (e.g. the ankle).

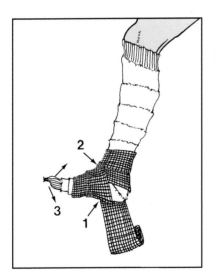

70. Application (c): Ensure the limb is correctly positioned, and apply each turn so that it overlaps the one beneath by half a width (1). It is permissible to use a figure-of-eight (2) round the ankle, elbow and knee to assist the bandage to lie neatly in conformity with the contours of the limb beneath. Turn back the stockingette (3) before applying the top layers of the bandage, and make quite certain that there will be no sharp or hard cast edges which can cause ulceration of the skin.

71. Application (d): In some cases close moulding of the cast may be encouraged by the temporary application of a firm external bandage. For this a thick cotton or crepe bandage may be used. This is first wetted, and then wrapped tightly round the limb. This will also be found helpful in retaining the last turn or two of the resin bandages, which often have a disturbing tendency to peel away before they set. Remove the wet overbandage once the cast has set.

72. Removal of resin casts: Because of their inherent springiness, resin casts cannot be cracked open after they have been cut down one side as can plasters. In most cases it is necessary to bivalve by cutting down both sides. In the case of leg casts, it is best to turn down the sole piece first. Either shears or an oscillating saw may be used; in the latter case, a dust extractor should be employed to avoid the inhalation of resin dust. Resin casts are less likely to break after windowing than plasters.

73. Assessment of union (a): Union in a fracture cannot be expected until a certain amount of time has elapsed, and it is pointless to start looking too soon. (See individual fractures for guidelines.) When it is reasonable to assess union, the limb should be examined out of plaster. Persistent oedema at the fracture site suggests union is incomplete.

74. Assessment of union (b): Examine the limb carefully for tenderness. Persistent tenderness localised to the fracture site is again suggestive of incomplete union.

75. Assessment of union (c): Persistent mobility at the fracture site is certain evidence of incomplete union. Support the limb close to the fracture with one hand, and with the other attempt to move the distal part in both the anterior and lateral planes. In a uniting fracture this is not a painful procedure.

76. Assessment of union (d): Although clinical assessment is often adequate in many fractures of cancellous bone, it is advisable in the case of the shafts of the femur, tibia, humerus, radius and ulna to have up-to-date radiographs of the region. The illustration is of a double fracture of the femur at 14 weeks. In the proximal fracture, the fracture line is blurred and there is external bridging callus of good quality; union here is fairly far advanced. In the distal fracture, the fracture line is still clearly visible, and bridging callus is patchy. Union is incomplete, and certainly not sufficient to allow unprotected weight bearing.

In assessing radiographs for union, be suspicious of unevenly distributed bridging callus, of a persistent gap, and of sclerosis or broadening of the bone ends. Note that where a particularly rigid system of internal fixation has been employed, bridging callus may be minimal or absent, and endosteal callus may be very slow to appear.

If in doubt regarding the adequacy of union, continue with fixation and re-examine in 4 weeks.

Note that in all cases you must assess whether the forces the limb is exposed to will result in displacement or angulation of the fracture, or cause such mobility that union will be prevented: you must balance the following equation:

External forces < (degree of union + support supplied by any internal fixation device and/ or external splintage).

CHAPTER

4

Open fractures: internal fixation

1. Open fractures: immediate care: When the case first presents, ensure that the following procedures are carried out in every case: (1) Take a bacteriology swab from the wound. (2) Commence a short course of appropriate antibiotics (see p. 50). (3) Cover the wound with care, using sterile dressings (to reduce the risks of secondary (hospital) infection). (4) Apply temporary splintage (e.g. a plaster back shell, or if appropriate, an inflatable splint).

2. Type I, technically open fractures: (1) The risks of infection are slight and are unlikely to be lessened by wide exposure (although this is advocated by some). The wound should be thoroughly cleaned (2) and a sterile dressing applied locally (3). Thereafter the method of supporting the fracture must be decided (see p. 80 and also Regional Injuries). If a plaster cast is being applied there *must* be allowance for swelling, e.g. by using a backshell or by splitting a cast applied over copious wool.

3. Type I, open from within out: The wound is small with clean or minimally bruised, viable edges (1). The skin edges may be minimally excised, and the wound extended (2) to allow a thorough inspection of the soft tissues and bone ends. It is unlikely that much will be required in the form of excision of contaminated or avascular tissue to achieve a thorough debridement. *Advantage may be taken of the exposure to allow an accurate open reduction of the fracture.*

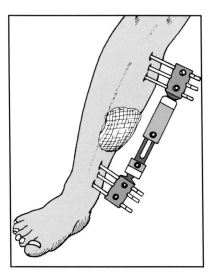

4. Type I ctd: Carry out a thorough (preferably pulsatile) wound lavage. Up to 10 L of normal saline may be used (followed by some with 2 L of bacitracin-polymyxin solution (1)). Primary closure of the skin is not advisable, but it may be helpful to use subcutaneous anchoring sutures (2) to prevent undue retraction and aid secondary suture. Apply a dressing which ensures the tissues remain moist (e.g. saline-soaked swabs over vaseline gauze). Attention must then be paid to fixation of the fracture.

5. Type I ctd: Inspect the wound after 48 hours; if necessary, perform any secondary debridement. If the wound remains clean, the aim should be to carry out a (delayed primary) wound closure under repeat antibiotic cover at 5 days (1). If the wound cannot be closed without tension, any remaining defect should be covered with a split-skin meshed graft (2) (which allows the escape of exudate). If the wound is dirty, then it should be treated by radical excision of all necrotic and infected tissue every 2–3 days until clean and ready to be grafted.

6. Type II open fractures: These should be managed along similar lines. *In Type III* injuries perform a rigorous lavage and debridement (with, if needed, wound enlargement): all foreign material must be removed along with any completely devitalised tissue (including small bone fragments). The wound should be left open dressed, or a vacuum dressing applied. To facilitate wound management (conducted as in Frame 5) an external fixator or locked intramedullary nail may be the best way to hold the fracture.

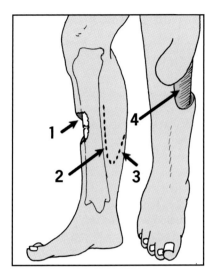

7. Type III *ctd:* If bone is exposed, the aim should be to get it covered within 5 days, to reduce the risks of secondary infection, and the initial application of a negative pressure dressing is usually advised. Split skin grafts will only survive if applied to a vascular bed, so that they cannot be used over open joints, bone devoid of periosteum, and tendons without paratenon. Thought must be given to future access (e.g. for bone grafting should union fail). In these circumstances other methods of cover must be employed. These should only be undertaken by a surgeon experienced in plastic surgical techniques,

and *consultation with a plastic surgeon prior to the initial procedure,* with later transfer to a Plastic Surgical Unit is highly desirable.

The local fascio-cutaneous flap: This is the commonest and most useful technique. These flaps include skin and fascia, but not muscle. (Skin flaps in the lower limb which do not include the fascial layer have a poor record of success.) Distally-based flaps are sometimes used to cover defects in the distal third of the leg. Careful planning of the flap is required. In the example (left) of the defect (1) to be covered, the anterior limb (2) of the flap to be raised is placed 1–2 cm posterior to the posteromedial border of the tibia. The posterior limb (3) may cross the midline. After the flap has been raised and swung (4), the resulting defect is covered with split skin grafts.

8. Type III *ctd:* Other plastic surgical techniques include the following:

Muscle flaps: These are generally reliable, but may result in functional loss.
(i) The gastrocnemius myocutaneous flap: this particularly proves good cover round the knee and in the proximal third of the tibia. Either the medial or lateral head may be used. (The muscle belly is isolated from soleus, its attachment to the Achilles tendon divided, and it is freed from its other head before the flap is swung.)
(ii) The soleal myocutaneous flap: this may be used for cover in the middle third of the tibia. (The muscle is detached 1 cm distal to

its musculotendinous junction, transposed, and anchored distally.) Added length may be obtained by making several transverse incisions in its sheath. At a suitable time, its outer surface may be covered with split skin grafts.

Free microvascular flaps: the commonest and most useful sources are from the latissimus dorsi or rectus abdominis. The techniques are highly specialised, and careful planning must extend to dealing with the secondary defect. Failure is generally due to vascular problems or infection at the recipient site.

Where bone grafting is required this should be carried out as soon as it is safe to do so. *In the case of Type I and Type II open fractures,* this can be considered 2–3 weeks after wound healing. *In the case of Type III open fractures,* grafting should be delayed for 6 weeks after healing has been obtained. Where there is extensive bone loss, future reconstruction may be possible using an Ilizarov bone transport technique.

Type IIIc open fractures have the highest failure and amputation rate, due to vascular difficulties or infection. In handling these cases the fracture must be soundly fixed and any arterial repair (e.g. by an interpositional graft) achieved within 4–6 hours; the vascular problem should be dealt with by an experienced vascular surgeon, and not delegated. Prophylactic fasciotomies should be carried out.

9. Degloving injuries (a): Here an extensive area of skin is torn from its underlying attachments and thereby deprived of its blood supply. In the hand or arm it is commonly caused by the limb being crushed between rollers (1), the so-called wringer injury; in the leg, trunk or pelvis it may result from the shearing effect of a vehicle wheel in a run-over accident.

10. Degloving injuries (b): The skin may remain unbroken (closed injury, 2 in Frame 9), when the limb feels like a fluid-containing bag, due to an extensive haematoma between the skin and fascia. Such injuries are sometimes missed. If the skin is torn (open injury, 3 in Frame 9), this creates a large flap of full-thickness skin when the wound may be extensively ingrained with road dirt. The skin itself may in some cases appear quite normal, with perhaps some central bruising, while in others it may be flayed. In either case, massive sloughing is likely although some proximally based flaps have a modest chance of viability.

Treatment Controversy exists in the treatment of these comparatively uncommon but serious injuries. It is agreed that if nothing is done in closed injuries that the skin will undergo necrosis. If the floating skin is excised as is normally advised, a large defect will result, and the aim should be for its immediate cover. In the thigh, split skin grafts may be used, and if the degloved skin shows little evidence of surface damage it may be employed, with the grafts being harvested before the skin is excised; in other cases the grafts may be taken from elsewhere (e.g. the other thigh).

Split skin grafts lack resistance to trauma, but full thickness skin is less likely to take; and if large areas are involved there may be problems with drainage and exudate lifting the graft from its bed, giving a poor result. Those who prefer using full thickness skin, because of particular circumstances or from personal choice, often de-fat the skin (to lower its oxygen demands), to fenestrate it (to let it go further and permit the passage of exudate), and to use a vacuum system (to improve local blood supply, improve graft adherence and facilitate drainage). Where there is a proximally based flap with apparent viability it may be sewn back, perhaps after defatting, and with good drainage. In some situations (e.g. the foot and achilles tendon area, tibial shaft fractures, and the pelvis and perineum), and in secondary management, certain plastic surgical procedures such as rotational and free microvascular flaps may be required.
In any open injury it is vital to keep in mind the risks of serious, life-threatening infections, particularly tetanus and gas gangrene, and the appropriate protective measures must be taken.

11. PRINCIPLES OF INTERNAL FIXATION AND COMMON FIXATION METHODS

When it is intended to implant materials for the treatment of fractures, the following criteria must be satisfied:

1. **Freedom from tissue reaction**: It is self-evident that if foreign material is being implanted in the tissues it should be biologically inert, and not give rise to toxic reactions, local inflammatory changes, fibrosis, foreign body giant cell reactions, etc., which in turn are likely to produce local pain, swelling and impairment of function. There is evidence of an extremely low but apparently clear incidence of local, and possibly distal, metal-induced neoplasia. In consequence, in the younger patient (under 40 years), internal fixation devices are removed routinely once they have served their purpose.

2. **Freedom from corrosion:** Implanted materials should not corrode. Where stainless steel is used it should be of an accepted grade and free from impurities; steps should be taken to avoid the initiation of corrosion problems by fretting occurring at the point of contact between the separate components of an implant. It is essential to avoid electrolytic degradation, and in practice this means that if more than one implant is used at the same side (e.g. a plate and screws) that identical materials are employed.

3. **Freedom from mechanical failure:** Implants must satisfy the purposes for which they are intended. To withstand the forces to which they will be subjected demands a satisfactory compromise between the materials used and the design of the implant. In the treatment of fractures, implants generally must have great mechanical strength in association with small physical bulk; consequently most are made of metal. Of the suitable metals, the most frequently employed are: (1) certain stainless steels, (2) alloys of chromium, cobalt and molybdenum (e.g. Vitallium®, Vinertia®), (3) titanium. The chrome-cobalt alloys are biologically very inert, but are difficult to machine so that most implants, including screws, are microcast using the lost wax technique; this adds to their cost. The stainless steels are less inert, but are easier to machine and are cheaper. In the case of titanium, the favourable combination of high strength, light weight, high fatigue strength, low modulus of elasticity and relative inertness, allows the fabrication of thinner plates and stronger intramedullary nails. It also produces fewer artefacts in CT and MRI scans, allowing, for example, earlier and better detection of avascular necrosis in femoral neck fractures.

In certain situations other materials are sometimes used; e.g. in fractures of the femur in the region of the stems of hip replacements it is possible to employ nylon cerclage straps to facilitate stability. At the ankle, biodegradable plastic dowels may be used to treat certain malleolar fractures, and have the advantage that their slow absorption obviates any need for their later removal. Sensitivity to these implants (in the form of a low grade inflammatory response) is, however, a not uncommon occurrence. Where it is desirable to have a certain amount of flexibility in a plate to encourage the formation of some external bridging callus, carbon fibre plates are sometimes used.

Fixation devices and systems Fractures vary enormously in pattern; bones vary in their size, texture and strength. To cope with even the most common situations and be a match for every subtle variation of circumstance requires an impressive range of devices and instruments for their insertion. The design of fixation devices has in the past been somewhat haphazard, and aimed at the treatment either of one fracture or the solution of a single fixation problem. There have been attempts to produce integrated systems of fracture fixation: sets of devices which can contend with any fracture situation. The most outstanding system, now firmly established, is that developed by the Association for the Study of Internal Fixation [ASIF or AO (Arbeitgemeinschaft für Osteosynthesefragen)]. (This group of general and orthopaedic surgeons was founded in 1956 by Maurice E. Müller to research certain concepts propounded by Robert Danis.) As a result of their work, apart from the development of a series of screws, plates and other devices, and the corresponding instrumentation, the Association is responsible for some change in emphasis in the philosophy of fracture treatment. They feel that the common aim, a return to full function in the shortest time, can often best be achieved by the use of internal fixation devices, of such strength and design that external splintage can frequently be discarded permitting immediate joint freedom, early weight bearing, short-term hospitalisation, and early return to work and other activities. These ideals are often achieved, but it must be stressed that optimum results cannot be obtained without the necessary technical knowledge of the system and a degree of mechanical aptitude, both of which can be acquired by appropriate training and experience.

With any form of internal fixation great importance must always be placed on recognising which cases are best treated in this way. It is equally important to recognise which cases are not suited to treatment by internal fixation, and those which may be dealt with either surgically or conservatively.

It is in the last group that there is often some difficulty, and it is important to remember the hazards of infection; even though it may be uncommon, it must always be a feared complication which on occasion can turn a comparatively minor fracture into a disaster. In certain situations the risks of infection may be reduced and fracture fixation achieved by using minimally invasive techniques (such as closed intramedullary nailing). Disturbance of the fracture haematoma is best avoided if at all possible as this may delay or prevent union; the risks may be reduced by the use of Wave or Less Invasive Plate Systems (see p. 77).

As in many branches of surgery, the core problem is in deciding how many excellent results are required to balance the occasional serious failure, and the compromise to be made between the particulars of a case and the outlook and judgement of the surgeon.

12. Principles of internal fixation and common devices: Cortical bone screws (a): The AO cortical bone screw enjoys widespread use and is probably the commonest of all internal fixation devices. The standard screw has an outside diameter of 4.5 mm (1) and a core diameter of 3.0 mm (2). The thread form is a modified buttress (3), of 1.75 mm pitch (circa 15 TPI). The large head has a hemispherical undersurface (4) and contains a hexagon socket (5) which is used for its insertion.

13. Cortical bone screws (b): To insert an AO screw, the bone is drilled with a 3.2 mm drill (1), preferably using a guide to maintain its perpendicularity. The hole is then tapped (2) and sized, so that the correct length of screw (from a wide range) can be chosen. This is then inserted using a hex screwdriver (3). In certain circumstances it is necessary to use smaller screws (e.g. in dealing with phalangeal fractures) and screws of 3.5, 2.7, 2 and 1.5 mm are available in the AO range.

14. Cortical bone screws (c): When two bone fragments are being approximated with a screw, it is usually desirable to do so in such a manner that the adjacent surfaces are compressed one against the other – this improves the quality of the fixation, reduces the risks of non-union, and may be essential if the fracture will otherwise be unsupported (e.g. if a cast is not being applied). To do this, a clearance (or gliding) hole is drilled in the nearest fragment; tightening the screw draws the two fragments together: the so-called lag screw principle.

15. Cortical bone screws (d): *Placing the screws.* Two mutually exclusive screw positionings may be used: (i) to obtain the most effective compression, and to avoid side thrusts which might displace the alignment of bone fragments, screws should be inserted at right angles to the plane of the fracture (1); (ii) to offer the maximum resistance to torsional forces, screws should be inserted at right angles to the cortex (2). In practice, a combination of these two placements may be employed with effect (3).

16. Cortical bone screws (e): In long bones, one or more screws may be used to hold a fracture in perfect alignment (Illus.). Such an arrangement can seldom suffice without additional support: this may be in the form of plaster cast, but commonly a plate is used to neutralise any torsional or bending stresses that the fracture might be subjected to (neutralising plate). Note that if the stresses are great (e.g. unsupported weight bearing) that some of the load *must* be carried by the bone, otherwise eventual fatigue fracture of the plate is likely.

17. Cancellous bone screws (a): Screws designed for insertion in cancellous bone have a coarse pitch and a narrow thread angle, a combination which at its extremes produces auger forms. *AO cancellous bone screws* (with diameters of 6.5 or 4 mm) may be *partially threaded* (for use as lag screws) (1), or *fully threaded* (2) (when used to fix plates in the metaphyseal regions of long bones). The near cortex only is usually threaded, the screw cutting its own path in the cancellous bone (3).

In demanding situations with multiple casualties, the principles of dealing with war wounds in the field may apply. These include thorough wound debridement and drainage, immobilisation, and delayed wound coverage or closure. External fixation, Kirschner wires, plaster casts and traction may be used to provide skeletal stability and aid soft tissue healing in preference to the use of internal fixation procedures.

Factors affecting healing; complications; pathological fractures

FACTORS AFFECTING THE RATE OF HEALING OF A FRACTURE

1. TYPE OF BONE

Cancellous bone (spongy bone) Healing in cancellous bone is generally well advanced 6 weeks from the time of the injury, and protection of the fracture can almost invariably be abandoned by that time. This applies to fractures of bones which are composed principally of cancellous tissue, and also to fractures involving the cancellous bone to be found at the ends of long bones. This rule is illustrated in the following examples:

1. Weight bearing after a fracture of the calcaneus may be permitted after about 6 weeks.
2. A patient with a traumatic wedge fracture of a vertebral body may commence full mobilisation after 6 weeks.
3. Plaster fixation may be discarded after 5–6 weeks following a Colles fracture of the wrist.
4. Weight may be allowed through the leg 6 weeks after a fracture of the tibial plateau.
5. Bed rest for 6 weeks is usually advised for any fracture of the pelvis involving those parts through which weight transmission is mediated.

Cortical bone (Compact bone) Endosteal callus may take many months to become reasonably well established, and many uncomplicated long bone fractures may take 9–18 weeks to unite. In some cases, however, abundant external bridging callus may allow an earlier return of function. For example:

1. The average time to union of a fracture of the tibial shaft treated conservatively is 16 weeks.
2. Fractures of the humeral shaft can often be left unsupported after 10 weeks.
3. On the other hand, fractures of the metatarsals, metacarpals and phalanges, where external bridging callus is usually substantial, are usually quite firm in 4–5 weeks.

2. PATIENT AGE

In children, union of fractures is rapid. The speed of union decreases as age increases until skeletal maturity is reached. There is then not a great deal of difference in the rate between young adults and the elderly. For example, in a child, union may be expected in a fractured femur a little after the number of weeks equivalent to its numerical age have passed: viz. a fractured femur in a child of 3 years is usually united after 4 weeks; a fractured femur in a child of 8 years is usually sound after 9 weeks. In contrast, a fracture of the femoral shaft in an adult may take 3–6 months to unite.

Apart from great rapidity of union it should be noted that children have remarkable powers of remodelling fractures. These powers are excellent as far as displacement is concerned, and are often good for slight to moderate angulation. Remodelling is poor in the case of axial rotation in both adults and children. The power to remodel decreases rapidly once adolescence is reached and epiphyseal fusion is imminent.

3. MOBILITY AT THE FRACTURE SITE

Excessive mobility persisting at the fracture site (due, for example, to poor fixation) may interfere with vascularisation of the fracture haematoma; it may lead to disruption of early bridging callus and may prevent endosteal new bone growth. One of the main aims of all forms of internal and external splintage is to reduce mobility at the fracture site, and hence encourage union. Absolute rigidity, however, may discourage external callus formation, so that reliance is placed on the internal fixation device – typically a plate – until the long process of endosteal union is complete. Nevertheless, if splintage is inadequate, union may be delayed or prevented.

4. SEPARATION OF BONE ENDS

Union will be delayed or prevented if the bone ends are separated, for this interferes with the normal mechanisms of healing. (The converse is also true, namely that compression of the fracture facilitates union.) Separation may occur under several circumstances:

1. **Interposition of soft tissue between the bone ends.** For example, in fractures of the femoral shaft, one of the bone ends may become isolated from the other by herniating through some of the surrounding muscle mass, thereby delaying or preventing union. Fractures of the medial malleolus may fail to unite due to infolding of a layer of periosteum between the fragments.

2. **Excessive traction.** Excessive traction employed in the maintenance of a reduction may lead to separation of the bone ends and non-union. This may occur, for example, in femoral shaft fractures, particularly those treated by skeletal traction.

3. **Following internal fixation.** In some situations where internal fixation is used to hold a fracture, absorption of bone may occur at the fracture site; the fixation device may continue to hold the bone fragments in such a way that they are prevented from coming together; and mechanical failure may ensue. A bulky internal fixation device may in itself interfere with the local blood supply and the fracture haematoma. Where possible, steps should be taken to avoid this (e.g. by using a LISS plate with locking screws and a minimally invasive technique).

5. BONE LOSS

This is comparatively rare, with the tibia and femur being most commonly affected; even less common is significant loss in the humerus and forearm bones. The main causes are bone extrusion in open fracture at the site of the causal incident or during transport, bone removal occurring during debridement procedures, and injuries due to gunshots or explosions. Loss most commonly affects the diaphysis; loss of metaphyseal or articular bone is generally associated with high-energy dissipation injuries.

If the loss is substantial then treatment will be prolonged and difficult, and because of the mechanism of injury many of these cases have accompanying problems with skin loss, tissue contamination, and accompanying neural and vascular damage. Other factors such as the patient's age and medical state, and other injuries will influence the management of the case. The first decision that must be made is therefore whether amputation is the best approach. This is not always easy, and the general view is that this must be decided on a completely individual assessment of the factors involved. While

1. Supracondylar fracture of humerus with soft tissue between bone ends.

use of the Mangled Extremity Severity Index (see p. 51) may help in taking all the important factors into account, it has been shown to be somewhat unreliable in evaluating those cases where it indicates that amputation should be performed.

Where it has been decided not to amputate, an appropriate method of fixation of the fracture must be chosen. The procedure to be adopted depends on the site and extent of the bone loss, and other local factors. In the femur, tibia and humerus (unless there is any contraindication), locked intramedullary nails generally give the best support for losses up to 6 cm, and at the later stages, with the newer devices, may allow bone lengthening procedures to be carried out. Autogenous bone grafting may also be required. In the forearm, and also in the case of the humerus, plates and screws are usually employed. External fixators may also be used, although unilateral frames do not give sufficient support where there is a significant segmental defect in the leg. In this case, the Ilizarov and other circular frames are of particular value, especially when subsequent bone lengthening is planned, and may be employed where the defect exceeds 6 cm.

The general approach is to fix the fracture at its true length, paying particular attention to rotation. However, where the skin poses a problem it is often useful to allow initial shortening of the limb while aiming to correct this later with a subsequent limb lengthening procedure.

There are many other approaches to dealing with the vagaries of these injuries. These include calcium phosphate cement which may be used for small metaphyseal or calcaneal defects; allografts, particularly in young patients with loss of a portion of a joint surface; vascularised fibular grafts, especially in the forearm; the creation of a one-bone forearm or lower leg; the use of bone substitutes and bone growth factors; and joint replacement procedures where there is a substantial loss of articular surfaces.

6. INFECTION

Infection in the region of a fracture may delay or prevent union. This is especially the case if, in addition, movement is allowed to occur at the fracture. Infection of the fracture site is extremely rare in conservatively treated closed fractures; infection, if it occurs, follows either an open injury or one treated by internal fixation. Where infection becomes well established in the presence of an internal fixation device, it is often difficult to achieve healing without removal of the device which acts as a foreign body and a nidus for persisting infection. This is especially the case if there is breakdown of the overlying skin and the establishment of a sinus. Not infrequently the situation arises where cast fixation alone is unable to provide the degree of fixation necessary for union if the device is removed, and where infection is likely to remain if it is not. In such circumstances it is usually wiser to retain the fixation device until union is reasonably well advanced, or to consider using an external fixator. In some cases where sound healing can be obtained and maintained after removal of an internal fixation device, it may be possible to repeat the internal fixation in the sterile environment that has been obtained.

MRSA Infections. Established infections with methicillin-resistant staphylococcus aureus may pose enormous problems: for the patient, in extreme cases, with risk of life, and in others to the prolongation of treatment and inferior results; for surgeons and nursing staff, with difficulties in

2. Chronic bone infection and failure of union of tibia following plating (plate removed).

management; and overall, with the greatly increased cost implications. The extent of the problem and the procedures adopted to deal with it vary from country to country, but many measures are common to all. In the UK, Giannoudis and others[1] suggest the following protocol for the identification of MRSA carriers, and the treatment of an established infection.

1. Strict adherence to national guidelines for screening in high-risk areas with:
   (a) Screening on admission for all regional/national referral centres, while high-risk areas should screen the following patients: those known to be previously affected or colonised; frequent re-admissions; those transferred from MRSA-infected wards or nursing homes; and those transferred from hospital abroad.
   (b) Discharge screening.
   (c) Screening of the nose, perineum, skin lesions and manipulated sites of all other patients after a single case has been detected.
   (d) Isolation of carriers.
   (e) Screening of all staff if additional cases occur.
   (f) Isolation of patients before negative swab results have been received. On identification of positive swab cultures for MRSA, the patients should be kept in isolation.
2. Treatment of carriers as outlined in the national guidelines with:
   (a) The use of nasal muciprocin for 5 days, repeated if further swabs show persistent colonization.
   (b) Bathing in antiseptic detergents such as 4% chlorhexidine or 2% triclosan for patients carrying MRSA at any site. This may be repeated if the strain is not eradicated.
   (c) Application of hexachlorophane powder to the axilla and groin, if they are thought to be colonized.
   (d) Treatment of throat carriers is not required but, if undertaken, this normally requires systemic treatment with rifampicin and fusidic acid, or ciprofloxacin.
3. Administration for 5 days of nasal muciprocin in combination with a triclosan bath on the day of surgery to all patients scheduled to receive implanted prosthetic material.
4. Education of nursing and medical staff on hand hygiene which is effective, although compliance is poor.
5. Treatment of an established infection initially with vancomycin while the patient is in hospital. Treicoplanin or linezolid can then be given on an out-patient basis. The length of administration should be decided by the treating clinician.

7. DISTURBANCE OF BLOOD SUPPLY

It is obvious that for the normal multiplication of bone cells and their precursors an adequate blood supply is required. Where the blood supply to an area is reduced, or where there is interference with the blood supply to both major fragments – e.g. in radionecrosis of bone – healing may be interfered with. On the other hand, reduction of the blood supply to one fragment, especially if cancellous bone is involved, may not interfere with union; indeed, in some situations it may apparently stimulate it. The most striking examples of this are fractures of the femoral neck and scaphoid, where the phenomenon of avascular necrosis is most frequently discovered in soundly united fractures. Interference with the blood supply to one fragment at the time of injury leads to immediate bone death; this is frequently followed by sound union of the fracture. Collapse of necrotic bone beyond the level of union is observed at a later date.

Again, a bulky internal fixation device may in itself interfere with the local blood supply and the fracture haematoma, delaying union. Where possible this should be avoided by choosing the most appropriate device.

8. PROPERTIES OF THE BONE INVOLVED

Fracture healing is also affected by a number of imperfectly understood factors which lead to variations in the speed of union. The clavicle is a spectacular example; non-union is extremely rare, the time to clinical union is unexcelled by any other part of the skeleton, yet movement at the fracture site cannot be controlled with any efficiency. Union of the tibia is often slow to a degree that is difficult to explain even when the influence of its nutrient artery and fracture mobility are taken into account.

9. OTHER FACTORS

1. **Effects of smoking.** Smoking has a deleterious effect on fracture union, often being a significant factor in the rate and quality of union.
2. **Joint involvement.** When a fracture involves a joint, union is occasionally delayed. This may be due to dilution of the fracture haematoma by synovial fluid.
3. **Bone pathology.** Many of the commonest causes of pathological fracture do not seem to delay union in a material way. (Union may progress quite normally in, for example, osteoporosis, osteomalacia, Paget's disease and most simple bone tumours.) Some primary and secondary malignant bone tumours may delay or prevent union (see pp 110–113).
4. **HIV/AIDS.** In humankind the HIV virus encodes its RNA within host cells, particularly CD4 (T-helper) lymphocytes, resulting in their depletion and an adverse effect on immunity. Effective retroviral therapy reduces the viral load in the serum and helps restore the CD4 cells. The level of these cells in the serum forms a valuable indicator of the severity of the infection and response to any treatment. Infections should be graded. This may be done on clinical grounds, using the four stages advocated by the World Health Organization, or by using a combination of clinical signs and CD4 levels (which results in 12 grades of severity) as described by the Centre for Disease Control and Prevention.

In closed fractures, and as a general rule, conservative methods of treatment are to be preferred wherever possible. Nevertheless, infections occurring in cases treated by internal fixation appear to be due mainly to contamination rather than an impaired immunity response, and open methods may be pursued so long as strict attention is paid to asepsis and careful tissue handling. Prophylactic antibiotics in the form of a first generation cephalosporin have been recommended by Harrison.[2]

In open fractures, if internal fixation is used, the rate of infection is often unacceptably high, and this line of treatment should be avoided where possible. In the case of the tibia an external fixator may be used, although an increase in pin-track infections should be anticipated. It need hardly be stated that in every case the strictest precautions must be taken to avoid the operator being exposed to the infected tissues and serum of the patient.

of a fracture or dislocation. In these cases, the circulation is immediately restored by correction of the deformity, and this should always be carried out as expeditiously as possible. In closed fractures other arterial disturbances are found, but these are relatively uncommon. A ragged bone edge may cause arterial rupture, leading to the rapid formation of a large haematoma. A fracture may also give rise to profound arterial spasm, aneurysm, or intimal stripping. In open fractures, arterial rupture often declares itself by the nature and the extent of the accompanying haemorrhage.

Diagnosis If the pulses distal to the injury site cannot be palpated, the patient should be resuscitated and reassessed within an hour. The most reliable guide to the situation is the Doppler pressure. To take this, a sphygmomanometer cuff should be positioned above the injury site and the Doppler signal located. The cuff is then inflated; the pressure at which the signal disappears is the Doppler pressure. Repeat the examination on the good side. If the pressures are not equal, the advice of a vascular surgeon should be sought *immediately*. If no Doppler equipment is available, then advice should be sought, again without delay, should the peripheral pulses on the injured side be reduced or absent. Angiography may be required, and is especially recommended after dislocations of the knee.

Treatment It is obvious that the survival of a useful limb is dependent on restoration of the circulation. Where this is not achieved by reduction of the fracture, exploration of the affected vessel is mandatory. Treatment is then dependent on the findings. If the artery is cleanly divided, an end-to-end anastomosis may be performed. In the presence of a deficit, an in-line reversed vein graft is often used. In either case, to prevent damage to the suture line, internal fixation of the fracture is an essential part of the procedure and is often performed first.

Most of the cases that appear to be due to arterial spasm are in fact associated with intimal damage. Opening of the vessel is necessary to elucidate this, although preliminary irrigation with papaverine is sometimes tried. If intimal damage is confirmed, resection of the affected segment with grafting may be required.

Arterial obstruction leading to muscle death and nerve palsy may also result from swelling within the muscle compartments of a limb (see below).

Compartment Syndromes Post-traumatic swelling may gradually compromise the circulation within a closed fascial compartment in a limb. If unchecked, there may be necrosis of the muscles and loss of function in the nerves contained in the compartment. The effects depend on the speed of onset of the increased pressure, its duration, and degree. (For example, in the anterior compartment of the leg, local haemorrhage, or oedema of muscles following trauma or overactivity, may lead to an inexorable rise of pressure beyond the systolic blood pressure. This will result in necrosis of the anterior compartment muscles, loss of conduction in the deep peroneal nerve, sensory disturbance in the foot and foot drop.)

The clinical findings most commonly found include:

- *Pain* out of proportion to the injury
- *Pain on passive movements* of the fingers or toes (where the muscles being stretched lie within the confines of the suspect compartment)
- Diffuse *tenderness* over the muscles of the compartment (and not just over a fracture)

- Distal *pallor*
- *Progressive paralysis* of the muscles within the compartment
- *Paraesthesia* and *loss of vibration sense* in the territory supplied by the nerves passing through the compartment
- Loss of any *pulse* which is dependent on any vessel passing through the compartment (but beware of false negatives from retrograde flow).

(Before considering the diagnosis of a compartment syndrome it is of course presumed that circulatory problems associated with *external* pressure will have been excluded, e.g. by the thorough splitting of all dressings and casts.)

Of the above findings, severe pain is the most outstanding feature. Confirmation of the diagnosis may be obtained by measuring the pressure within a suspect compartment, and this should be done as close to any fracture as possible for the most accurate results. This may be done using a simple needle technique, a slit catheter, a side-ported needle, or an electronic transducer-tipped catheter. The last would seem to give the most accurate results, and is good for continuous monitoring (which is particularly desirable in cases complicated by head injury). It is considered that when the intracompartmental pressure exceeds 30 mmHg then operative intervention is indicated. However, the measurement of differential pressure (the diastolic blood pressure minus the intracompartmental pressure) is to be preferred, and if this falls below 30 mmHg, fasciotomy is indicated. In the case of the fascial compartments of the hand, threshold pressures for intervention are lower, being in the order of 15–20 mmHg.

Treatment It is vital that this is performed with great urgency and is by means of a fasciotomy which is extensive enough to completely relieve pressure build-up within the compartment concerned. In some cases it is advisable to extend fasciotomy to any adjacent compartments which are also at risk of being compromised. *Prophylactic fasciotomies* should be considered in all open fractures of Grade II and above and in any severe crushing injury. (For further details see under the appropriate regional sections.)

Immediate neurological disturbance Neurological complications occurring immediately after fractures and dislocations are comparatively uncommon. Nevertheless, in certain situations a nerve may be stretched over a bone edge in a displaced fracture, or over a bone end in a dislocation. If prolonged this will lead to local ischaemia and interruption of nerve conduction. If stretching is more severe there may be rupture of axons or of neural tubes: actual nerve division is rare, being seen mainly in association with open injuries (especially gunshot wounds). The commoner fractures and dislocations associated with nerve palsies include the following:

Injury	Nerve palsy
Dislocation of the shoulder	Axillary nerve palsy: rarely other brachial plexus lesions
Fracture of the shaft of the humerus	Radial nerve palsy
Dislocation of the elbow	Ulnar nerve palsy; sometimes median nerve affected
Fractures round the elbow	Median nerve palsy; less commonly, ulnar nerve, or posterior interosseous nerve
Dislocation of the hip	Sciatic nerve palsy
Dislocation of the knee or rupture of lateral ligament of the knee and fracture of medial tibial plateau	Common peroneal nerve palsy

Treatment The majority of nerve lesions are in continuity. Assuming that the fracture or dislocation has been reduced, recovery often begins after 6 weeks, progressing quite rapidly thereafter. *The skin* must be protected during the recovery period against friction, burns and other trauma so long as sensation remains materially impaired. *The joints* should be exercised passively to avoid stiffness. *Deformity* due to overactivity of unaffected muscles should be prevented: this applies particularly to the drop wrist of radial palsy, and the drop foot where the sciatic or common peroneal nerves are involved. Lively splintage may be particularly helpful in these circumstances. (Lively splints are splints which are hinged to permit movement, often while still supplying support, and generally have a spring incorporated against which the patient can work. For example, a lively wrist splint is hinged at the wrist which is thereby held in dorsiflexion by a tension spring on its dorsal surface. The patient can then repeatedly flex the wrist to exercise it against this resistance.)

Where there is a nerve palsy accompanying a fracture which is going to be treated surgically, opportunity may be taken to inspect the affected nerve. This will often help in establishing a prognosis, and may also permit definitive treatment of the injury (e.g. by removing any local pressure on the nerve). In the case of fractures of the humeral shaft accompanied by radial nerve palsy, primary open reduction, inspection of the nerve, and compression plating has been advocated in preference to conservative management of the fracture and expectant treatment of the palsy.

When an expected recovery does not occur, electromyography (EMG) and nerve conduction studies may be of occasional diagnostic value, but exploration is often required. Some also advocate a more aggressive approach in dealing with nerve palsies accompanying fracture, advising an EMG at 3 weeks, with exploration at 6 weeks if there is no change in a second EMG performed at that time.

In the case of nerve injury complicating a fresh injury, primary suture should be undertaken if the risks of infection are judged to be slight and facilities are good. Otherwise the nerve ends should be approximated with radio-opaque sutures or markers, and elective repair delayed until sound wound healing has been obtained. If nerve repair is not possible, reconstructive surgery or orthotic support of the paralysed part may be required.

Delayed neurological disturbance Sometimes a nerve palsy gradually develops long after a fracture has healed.

Tardy ulnar nerve palsy. This is the most striking example of this process. In a typical case the patient gradually develops over a period of a few months an ulnar nerve palsy which may become complete. The injury responsible is usually a supracondylar fracture or a Monteggia fracture–dislocation. The striking feature is the interval between the fracture and the nerve palsy. It is usually in the order of several years, and indeed may be as much as 60.

In a number of these cases there is a cubitus valgus deformity, and the resultant stretching of the nerve is usually regarded as being responsible for the onset of the palsy. Nevertheless, tardy ulnar nerve palsy also occurs in the presence of cubitus varus, so that progressive ischaemia of the nerve has come to be considered as another possible factor.

Treatment Tardy ulnar nerve palsy is usually treated by early transposition of the ulnar nerve. (The nerve is mobilised from its exposed position behind the medial epicondyle, brought round to the front of the elbow, and buried in the flexor muscles of the forearm just beyond their point of origin.)

Median nerve palsy Signs of median nerve compression may gradually develop a few months after a Colles fracture of the wrist. This is generally akin to the partial nerve lesions seen in the carpal tunnel syndrome. Some residual displacement of the fracture may reduce the space available in the carpal tunnel leading to pressure on the nerve and an incomplete palsy.

Treatment Symptoms are usually relieved by carpal tunnel decompression (by dividing the flexor retinaculum).

DELAYED TENDON RUPTURE This uncommon fracture complication is seen most frequently at the wrist, when after a Colles fracture, a patient loses the ability to extend the terminal joint of the thumb. This is due to rupture of the extensor pollicis longus tendon some weeks or months after the fracture. The rupture may result from the gradual fraying of the tendon as it rubs against the healing fracture, or it may be caused by traumatic or fibrotic interference with its arterial blood supply, resulting in local sloughing of the tendon.

Treatment In the case of the thumb, the best results are obtained by transposition and suture of the tendon of extensor indicis to the distal segment of extensor pollicis longus.

Visceral complications

1. Rupture of the urethra or bladder and perforation of the rectal wall may complicate fractures of the pelvis.
2. Rupture of the spleen, kidney or liver may follow severe local trauma, abdominal compression or crushing (such as, for example, run-over injuries).
3. Rupture of the intestines or tearing of the mesenteric attachments may also follow abdominal compression.
4. Paralytic ileus is occasionally seen following fractures of the pelvis and lumbar spine, the most likely cause being disturbance of the autonomic control of the bowel from retroperitoneal haematoma. Distension of the abdomen, absent or faintly tympanitic bowel sounds and vomiting are the usual features. It is, of course, imperative to exclude the possibility of perforation, especially when there is a history of a run-over injury. The diagnosis may be made on the basis of the history and clinical findings, but plain radiographs of the abdomen, abdominal paracentesis, an ultrasound examination, laparoscopy or laparotomy may be necessary where there is a history of direct injury. Treatment is by:
   (i) Nasogastric suction
   (ii) Intravenous fluids – the quantity and proportions being determined by the amount of aspirate and other losses, and serum electrolyte estimations. In the majority of cases, bowel sounds return within 36 hours, and intravenous fluids and suction may be discontinued shortly afterwards.
5. The cast syndrome: Abdominal distension and vomiting sometimes occur in patients being treated in plaster jackets, hip spicas, or plaster beds,

13. Paralytic ileus secondary to pelvic fracture: note the air distension of bowel loops in this plain abdominal film.

especially if the spine is hyperextended. When the onset is extremely rapid leading to shock and prostration, the superior mesenteric artery or cast syndrome may be suspected (i.e. there is a high intestinal obstruction due to duodenal compression by the superior mesenteric artery).

Treatment
  (i) If a plaster jacket has been applied, it should be removed. A patient being nursed in a plaster bed should be transferred to an ordinary bed or a Stryker frame.
 (ii) A large-bore gastric tube should be passed.
(iii) Fluid replacement therapy may be required.

Osteoarthritis See under causes of joint stiffness.

Implant complications
Mechanical effects Plates and intramedullary nails reduce the natural elasticity of the bone in the area that they lie. As a result, the loads to which a bone is subjected are not absorbed evenly throughout its length; stress concentrations tend to occur at the ends of internal fixation devices. In some cases this may lead to susceptibility to fracture which may occur with less violence than is needed in a normal bone. It is well known that after a plated fracture of the tibia has united, comparatively minor violence may result in a further fracture of the limb at either end of the plate. Similarly, after a minor fall on the side, the forces which would be absorbed by a normal femur may result in a fracture of the femoral neck in someone who has had an intramedullary nailing.

Corrosion No metal implant is completely inert, and the long-term risks of retention of implants within the body have not been fully evaluated. It is not uncommon for the tissues surrounding a stainless steel implant to become discoloured, with the formation of substantial masses of fibrous tissue. This is especially likely to occur if there has been fretting between components (e.g. between a plate and screw). There may be local aching pain, and this is an indication for removal of the device, assuming that the fracture is soundly healed.

The individual elements in the alloy that has been used for the fabrication of the implant may separate, giving rise to local toxic effects, and having the potential, once they enter the transport systems, of causing problems elsewhere. Stainless steel contains in the order of 13% chromium, and this element is well known for its local irritant effect and its potential for inducing sensitisation. Neoplasia has been reported in bone at the site of plates, and the implants have been considered as being responsible. It is possible that freed metal elements, after transportation, may be capable of causing neoplasia in the liver and elsewhere. Aluminium is used in certain other alloys used for implants; this is neurotoxic, competing with magnesium in the formation of tubulin, a primary structural protein in the nervous system: this mechanism has been linked with Alzheimer's disease.

Treatment While it must be stressed that problems of the above nature are rare, the risks of any long-term effects should be avoided where possible by the routine removal of implants once they have served their purpose; this is the general advice in patients under the age of 40 years. Over that age the indications are less powerful, but as a general rule intramedullary nails should be removed, as should any other device where there is evidence of local tissue reaction.

PATHOLOGICAL FRACTURES

A pathological fracture is one which has occurred in a bone which is abnormal or diseased.

In some cases the pathological process leads to progressive weakness of the bone so that fracture may occur spontaneously or after slight injury only. Fracture may occur as an inevitable event in some disease process, e.g. a fracture in the course of a destructive, chronic osteitis: always unwelcome, but causing no surprise. On the other hand, the disease process may be unknown to the patient and his practitioner, the trivial nature of the trauma giving concern to both.

Where bone strength is not materially impaired, the causal violence producing the fracture may not cause comment; in these circumstances the radiographs taken after the incident may give the first indication to anyone that something else is amiss. It follows that virtually any condition capable of being detected by radiographs of the skeleton may fall into this category – a limitless range of congenital, metabolic and neoplastic disease. Diagnosis as a result may be difficult, but fortunately there is one important point to take into consideration: where fracture is the presenting feature, the number of conditions commonly responsible is small. These include the following:

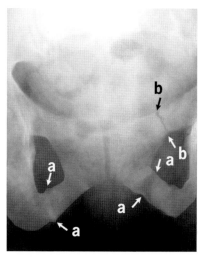

14. Osteoporosis: This is the commonest cause of pathological fracture, being especially important in the spine, the wrist and the femoral neck. It is most frequently due to lowering of hormone levels in association with age or the menopause: less frequently it follows disuse, rheumatoid arthritis or vitamin C deficiency which lead to a failure of osteoid tissue formation and the translucent appearance of bone on the radiographs. (Illus.: fracture of T6).

15. Osteomalacia (a): This is due to a failure in osteoid mineralisation and the radiographic appearances may be difficult to differentiate from osteoporosis. (Illus.: fracture of tibia and fibula.) It is usually secondary to an inability to utilise vitamin D (adult rickets) but is also seen where calcium is deficient in the diet (or excreted in renal acidosis), where phosphate is excreted in excess (Fanconi syndrome), or where vitamin D is not absorbed (e.g. steatorrhoea).

16. Osteomalacia (b): Stress fractures are common. Areas of bone translucency (Looser's zones) in the pelvis and long bones are characteristic. (Illus.: note changes in ischium (a) and pubic ramus fracture (b).) There are disturbances in the blood chemistry: the serum PO_4 is reduced, while the serum calcium is normal or reduced. Lowering of the mathematical product of the serum calcium and phosphate (in SI units) to less than 2.25 is generally confirmatory.

17. Osteomalacia (c): Occasionally a triradiate pelvis may be present and also be diagnostic. Osteomalacia may be treated with calciferol 1.25 mg per day, and calcium gluconate 1–2 g per day. The serum calcium, phosphate and urea should be monitored at regular intervals. Fracture healing is not materially impaired in either osteomalacia or osteoporosis.

18. Paget's disease (a): This common condition is frequently seen in association with fracture, particularly in the tibia and the femur. (Illus.: two healing fractures of the femur.) The radiological picture is complex, with frequently cyst formation, bone thickening, increased bone density and disturbances of bone texture. Stress fractures are common, and complete fractures are usually transverse.

19. Paget's disease (b): Increased bone density and deformity may in many situations make the use of internal fixation devices difficult. (Illus.: femoral neck fracture pinned in coxa vara: healing fracture of shaft.) The rate of healing and the soundness of bone union are not, however, usually greatly affected. In many situations conservative methods may be employed with success.

20. Paget's disease (c): Note that sarcomatous change (a) in this condition may be followed by fracture (b) as the cortical bone is eroded. Note, too, that the bone changes found in hyperparathyroidism and sometimes in metastatic disease may mimic Paget's disease.

21. Osteitis: Sudden collapse of bone secondary to infection is comparatively uncommon as a presenting feature, but is seen where the destructive processes are comparatively low grade. Thorough investigation and appropriate treatment is mandatory. (Illus.: Tuberculosis at the thoracolumbar level.)

22. Malignant bone tumours (a): The commonest malignant bone tumour is the metastatic deposit. Secondaries in bone occur most frequently from primary growths in lung or bronchus, breast, prostate or kidney. Any bone may be affected, but the spine, subtrochanteric region of the femur and the humeral shaft are amongst the commonest sites. (Illus.: metastatic deposit in humerus, primary in lung.)

23. Malignant bone tumours (b): Multiple myeloma in the pelvis (Illus.: with fracture of the femoral neck and a destructive lesion of the ilium) may sometimes be confused with secondary deposits from carcinoma of the prostate or other organs; full investigation is essential.

24. Malignant bone tumours (c): Primary malignant tumours of bone generally present with pain and swelling rather than fracture, but this is not always the case, especially perhaps in Ewing's tumour (Illus.: radiograph prior to fracture) and osteosarcoma. The aggressive, locally malignant osteoclastoma again usually presents with pain and swelling rather than fracture.

25. Malignant bone tumours (d): *Treatment:* Note the following points:
(a) Without treatment, union of a fracture occurring at the site of a malignant bone tumour seldom occurs.
(b) If the tumour is responsive to local radiotherapy or to chemotherapy, healing may occur with appropriate splintage, but will be slow.
(c) In the case of metastatic disease, internal fixation has much to recommend it unless the patient is moribund. Acrylic cement is sometimes used to reinforce a bone defect.
(d) In the case of primary malignant bone tumours, the occurrence of fracture may be a factor in some circumstances in the advocation of amputation.

26. Simple bone tumours and cysts (a): In the metacarpals, metatarsals (Illus.) and phalanges (Illus.), enchondromata are frequently encountered as a cause of pathological fracture. These are generally best treated by exploration, curettage and the packing of the resultant cavity in the bone with cancellous bone grafts.

27. Simple bone tumours and cysts (b): In children between the ages of 5 and 15 years, unicameral bone cyst is one of the most frequent causes of pathological fracture, especially in the proximal humeral shaft. The bone cortex may be thinned, but expansion is rare. The fracture should be treated conservatively. (If the fracture fails to heal and the cyst to disappear, curette and pack with bone grafts.)

28. Osteogenesis imperfecta: This hereditary disorder (dominant transmission) is characterised by bone fragility leading to bowing of the long bones, deformities of modelling, pathological fractures and stunting of growth. (Illus.: fracture of humerus with deformities of ribs.) Deafness and blue sclerotics are commonly associated. The condition generally declares itself in infancy

or childhood, but occasionally may not be diagnosed until skeletal demineralisation is noted later in life. Fracture healing is usually quite rapid, and most fractures may be treated successfully by conservative methods. Occasionally in the severer forms of this condition which present in childhood, internal fixation of the long bones by intramedullary nailing may be advocated as a prophylaxis against further fracture and to lessen bowing and other deformities of the legs.

Investigation of pathological fractures
Investigation of a pathological fracture may require some or all of the following:
1. A full personal and family history
2. Full clinical examination, including pelvic examination
3. Radiographs of the chest
4. Radiographs of the pelvis
5. Radiographs of the skull and skeletal survey
6. Estimation of the sedimentation rate and C-reactive protein
7. A full blood count, including a differential cell count
8. Estimation of the serum calcium, phosphate, serum Vitamin D, alkaline phosphatase and where appropriate, the acid phosphatase
9. Estimation of the serum proteins
10. Serum electrophoresis
11. Examination of the urine for Bence-Jones proteose
12. A bone scan
13. Marrow biopsy
14. Bone biopsy
15. Occasionally, radiographs of parents or sibs.

RECORDING AND COMMUNICATING: SOME SUGGESTED GUIDELINES

RECORDS

Careful note-taking in good patient management should already be recognised and practised, but in a field of medicine where evidence for insurance claims and litigation is commonly required, it is of particular importance. There are a number of areas where inadequacy is commonly found; these include the following:

1. Not infrequently when the handling of a case is being studied some time after the event, problems arise because entries or letters have been *undated*; and if, as is often the case, they are on separate sheets, the time that they have been made cannot be determined by their context. It is vital that any entry is clearly dated, and in the seriously ill patient whose condition is rapidly changing during the first few hours after admission, the *time* should be clearly stated as well.

2. Illegible handwriting is always a problem, but there should be no excuse for numerals and capital letters which are so badly formed that they cannot be read by others or even by the originator. When contractions are used (and these can be helpful in providing oases of upper-case meaningful clarity) only those in common use should be employed.

3. Paucity of notes (often very unfairly) suggests a similarly brief, and by implication, incomplete examination. In the heat of dealing with a seriously ill patient there is no time for detailed note-taking, but as soon as pressure eases, a full record should be made, and certainly this should be done *on the day of the admission*.

4. The interpretation of radiographs should be included in the notes, giving negative as well as positive findings. With the growing tendency to practise a degree of defensive medicine, radiographs should certainly be taken if there is any doubt about the nature or severity of an injury, and if radiographs are not taken, it is perhaps wise to say at the time why this has not been thought to be necessary.

5. If there is something that you are not sure of, indicate what this is (so that it cannot be claimed later that you had not considered it), and state the course you intend to take (with, if appropriate, the reasons for doing so).

TELEPHONING

Be clear whether the purpose of your call is to inform, to ask for advice, or to seek assistance: and have all the appropriate information at your fingertips. It is necessary to be able to describe a fracture patient in an unequivocal fashion, so that an unconfused picture of the problem is conveyed. There are undeniably different styles of doing this, but the following method is suggested:

1. Preamble
2. Precise fracture details
3. Particular qualifiers
4. Reason for call.

Preamble   After any niceties, including if necessary stating exactly who you are, give the age and sex of the patient along with any special attributes which bear directly on the reason for the call, e.g.:

> *'I have just admitted a 35-year-old man who is*
> *a professional ice skater. He has been in a road*

traffic accident and his main problem is ...' (Note that it is probably best to avoid contractions such as 'RTA' as they have to be translated, and may grate when used over the telephone.)

Precise fracture details The description of the fracture should always start with whether it is open or closed, and be followed by the bone involved and at what level; then the pattern of the fracture, and any displacement or angulation should be given, e.g.:

'... an open fracture of his right tibia in mid-shaft. It's a transverse fracture, but it's displaced medially and there's some lateral angulation. There's some shortening, and there's no bony contact.'

Particular qualifiers Where relevant these would include the following:

1. Complications of the local injury: this would include a description of the size, nature, location and potential contamination of a wound. It would also include details of any vascular or neurological problem.
2. Details of any other injuries sustained, e.g. other fractures, head injury, chest or abdominal injuries.
3. General condition of the patient, with, if appropriate, the time when he would be considered fit enough for anaesthesia and surgery.
4. Details of any treatment already carried out, e.g. fluid replacement, splintage, etc. For example:

'... The fracture is from within out, and the wound is 1 cm in length. It looks pretty clean, and there's no neurological or circulatory problem, and he has had no other injury. His general condition's fine; he seems to have had very little blood loss and his pulse and BP are OK. I've set up an IV line and put him in a back splint. He's not had anything by mouth for the last 6 hours. He's been seen by the anaesthetist who is happy to do him any time.'

Reason for call

1. When this is to inform only, the details of the treatment carried out and what is further proposed could, with profit, be expanded, e.g.:

'I'm planning to take him to theatre to debride the wound. I think I'll be able to get a good stable reduction under vision and I'll put the limb in plaster afterwards.'

2. When advice is sought, the nature of the problem should be clearly stated, e.g.:

'I think this fracture might do best if internally fixed, but I'm wondering whether this should be done right away, or whether I should just reduce it and splint it, and add it to the beginning of tomorrow's list.' (Not generally the best solution!)

3. When help is required, this should be clearly stated, e.g.:

> *'I think this is one you would want to treat by closed intramedullary nailing, and I've laid on theatre for seven thirty.'*

For suggestions on the making of follow-up notes, see Chapter 16, Fracture Clinics.

B

Regional injuries

6

The shoulder girdle and humerus

1. Clavicular injuries: mechanism of injury: Most (94%) clavicular injuries result from a direct blow on the point of the shoulder, generally from a fall on the side (A). Less commonly, force may be transmitted up the arm from a fall on the outstretched hand (B). Under the age of 30 years, road traffic and sporting injuries are the commonest causes. *Fracture:* The central 3/5 (1) is involved in about 2/3 of cases, and within this group fractures at the junction of the middle and outer thirds (2) are commonest. Fractures of the outer 1/5 (3) are much less common, and of the inner 1/5 (4) even less so. *Subluxations and dislocations:* These may involve the acromioclavicular joint (5) or the sternoclavicular joint (6). Fractures of the clavicle involving the acromioclavicular joint are uncommon (2.8% of cases).

2. Common patterns of fracture (a): Greenstick fractures are common, particularly at the junction between the middle and outer thirds. Fractures may not be particularly obvious on the radiographs and it is often helpful in children to have both shoulders included for comparison. The only abnormality visible in many cases is local kinking of the clavicular contours. Healing of this type of fracture is *rapid, and reduction is not required.*

3. Common patterns of fracture (b): In the adult, undisplaced fractures are also common, and are comparatively stable injuries. Late slipping is rare. Symptoms settle rapidly and minimal treatment is required.

4. Common patterns of fracture (c): With greater violence, there is separation of the bone ends. The proximal end under the pull of sternomastoid often becomes elevated (1). The shoulder loses the prop-like effect of the clavicle, so that it tends to sag downwards and forwards (2). Note (3) the glenoid, (4) the coracoid, (5) the acromion.

5. Common patterns of fracture (d): With greater displacement there is overlapping and shortening, but union is usually rapid. Remodelling, even in the adults, is so effective that strenuous attempts at reduction are unnecessary. Rare non-union is nevertheless seen most often in highly displaced fractures and those of the outer third. Pathological fracture may result from radionecrosis (following radiotherapy for breast carcinoma) and may be mistaken for a local recurrence.

6. Diagnosis: Clinically there is tenderness at the fracture site; sometimes there is obvious deformity with local swelling, and the patient may support the injured limb with the other hand. In cases seen some days after injury, local bruising is often a striking feature. Diagnosis is confirmed by appropriate radiographs; a single AP projection of the shoulder is usually adequate in the adult.

7. Treatment (a): The most important aspect of treatment is to provide support for the weight of the arm in which the clavicular tie has been impaired. As a rule this is best achieved with a broad arm sling (1). Additional fixation may be obtained by wearing the sling under the clothes (2). No other treatment is needed in greenstick or undisplaced fractures.

8. Treatment (b): Where there is marked displacement of a clavicular fracture an attempt to correct the anterior drift of the scapula round the chest wall (1) and improve the clavicular shortening is sometimes made. There is no simple way of achieving this. All methods attempt to apply pressure on the front of the shoulder (2) and although they are comparatively ineffective in terms of reduction, are helpful in reducing pain.

9. Treatment (c): Ring or Quoit method: Narrow gauge stockingette is cut into two lengths of about a metre each (1). The central portions are stuffed with cotton wool (2). One of the strips is taken and the padded area positioned over the front of the shoulder and tied firmly behind (3).

10. Treatment (d): The second strip is applied in a similar manner to the other shoulder (4). The patient is then advised to brace the shoulders back and the free ends of the ring pads are tied together (5). A pad of gamgee (a sandwich of cotton wool between layers of gauze) may be placed as a cushion beneath the knots (6).

11. Treatment (e): Figure-of-eight bandage: Pads of gamgee or cotton wool alone are carefully positioned round both shoulders (1). The patient, who should be sitting on a stool, is asked to brace back the shoulders; a wool roll bandage is then applied in a figure-of-eight fashion (2). For added security the layers may be lightly stitched together at the crossover (3).

12. Treatment (f): Commercially available clavicle rings, covered with chamois leather, may be applied and secured with a strap. Many other patterns of off-the-shelf clavicular supports are available. With all of these care must be taken to avoid pressure on the axillary structures and the additional support of a sling is desirable for the first 2 weeks or so. Note also that elderly patients tolerate clavicular bracing methods poorly, and sling support only may be advisable. (For internal fixation see Frame 25.)

13. Aftercare:
1. Clavicular braces of all types require careful supervision and, at least initially, may require inspection and possible tightening every 2–4 days.
2. Where braces are used in conjunction with a sling, the sling may usually be discarded after 2 weeks.
3. All supports may be removed as soon as tenderness disappears from the fracture site.
4. Physiotherapy is seldom required except in the elderly patient who has developed shoulder stiffness.
5. A child's mother should always be advised that the prominent callus round the fracture is a normal occurrence, and that it will disappear in a few months with remodelling.

Note: If there is evidence of *torticollis* accompanying a clavicular fracture, further investigation of the cervical spine is indicated, as this finding may indicate a coincidental injury at the C1–2 level (locked facet joints). If plain radiographs are insufficient to clarify the situation, a CT scan should if possible be carried out.

14. Acromioclavicular joint injuries: Injury to the acromioclavicular joint usually results from a fall in which the patient rolls on the shoulder. Note that the clavicle is normally attached to the scapula by (1) acromioclavicular, (2) conoid and (3) trapezoid ligaments. The scapular component of shoulder abduction requires free acromioclavicular movement.

15. Pathology: Note that: (1) in subluxations and sprains, damage is confined to the acromioclavicular ligaments, and the clavicle preserves some contact with the acromion. In dislocations (2) the clavicle loses all connection with the scapula, the conoid and trapezoid ligaments tearing away from the inferior border of the clavicle. The displacement may be severe, and the ensuing haematoma may ossify (3).

16. Diagnosis (a): The patient should be standing and the shoulders compared. The outer end of the clavicle will be prominent, and in cases of damage to the conoid and trapezoid ligaments the prominence may be quite striking. Local tenderness is always present.

17. Diagnosis (b): Confirm any subluxation by supporting the elbow with one hand gently pushing the clavicle down with the other. Improvement in the contour of the outer end of the clavicle will confirm the diagnosis of subluxation or dislocation.

92. Displaced fracture of greater tuberosity: These two-part injuries (Neer Group 4) may often be reduced by closed methods, but are liable to displace as the result of the unopposed action of the supraspinatus. It is probably best to internally fix these fractures, and this may be done with a single cancellous screw with a stress relieving washer under the head. This treatment is also indicated in Group I injuries where there is late displacement.

93. Two-part impacted fracture of the surgical neck: In the case illustrated there is minimal displacement and angulation showing in this single projection. These injuries may be treated conservatively with external supports (see Frame 95) and prolonged immobilisation is not necessary. Once pain has settled (usually after 2–3 weeks) mobilisation may be commenced.

94. Two-part unimpacted fracture of the surgical neck with slight angulation and/or displacement: In this Neer Group 1 injury an appreciable area of cancellous bone is in contact, generally assuring rapid healing. Secondary displacement is unlikely provided the limb has some initial protection (required anyway to relieve the severe pain which often accompanies these injuries). These may be internally fixed, but conservative management is usually adequate.

95. Conservative treatment of two-part fractures of the surgical neck (a): Slightly displaced and moderately angled humeral neck fractures may be treated satisfactorily by external support alone; many other fractures may be managed along similar lines. Firstly, the arm should be supported in a sling. Where disimpaction is undesirable (e.g. Frame 93) a broad arm sling is preferable (1). Where the fracture is disimpacted (e.g. Frame 94), then a collar and cuff sling (2) has some potential for gravitational correction of any angulation.

96. Conservative treatment (b): In addition, the arm should be protected from rotational stresses by a body bandage (e.g. of crepe bandages) (1) under the clothes (2). Alternatively, an expanding net support may be used (e.g. Netelast™) and this is certainly more comfortable in hot weather. Pain is often severe, and analgesics will be required in the first 1–2 weeks.

97. Conservative treatment (c): After 2 weeks the body bandage may be discarded unless pain is commanding. The sling should be worn under the outer clothes. The patient is advised to commence rocking movements of the shoulder (abduction, flexion (1)) and to remove the arm from the sling three or four times per day to flex and extend the elbow (2).

98. Conservative treatment (d): At 4 weeks the sling can be placed outside the clothes. Gentle active movements should be practised throughout the day. Over the next 2 weeks the patient should be encouraged to discard the use of the sling in gradual stages.

99. Conservative treatment (e): At 6 weeks the patient should be referred for physiotherapy if, as is usual, there is considerable restriction of movement. The range of movements (particularly glenohumeral; Illus.) should be recorded at fortnightly intervals, and physiotherapy discontinued when gains cease. Some permanent restriction of glenohumeral movement is common, but seldom incapacitating.

100. Two-part severely angled or displaced fractures of the surgical neck (a): (Neer Group 3). Open reduction and internal fixation is the treatment of choice for this pattern of injury in young and middle-aged adults. In the elderly patient a good result can be expected in these injuries when the deformity is accepted and conservative management is pursued along previously indicated lines. If the deformity is particularly severe or the patient very active, manipulative reduction should be attempted. (See Frames 105–107.)

101. Two-part fractures (b): There are several plates which have been designed specifically for this pattern of fracture. Some are anatomically pre-contoured, and many have the facility for using screws which lock into the plate. The Philos plate (Illus.) has a useful range of threaded holes and slots. It has plain holes for the use of Kirschner wires to temporarily hold the fragments in alignment.

102. Two-part fractures (c): In this example an anatomically contoured plate has been used to hold a fracture of the surgical neck which was initially severely displaced.

103. Two-part fractures (d): As an alternative to plates and screws an intramedullary nail with locking facilities may be used. The T2™ Proximal Humeral Nail (Illus.) is fabricated from titanium and is bent to allow a lateral entry point just medial to the tip of the greater tuberosity. Four screws can be inserted in the head (they are located by means of a jig), and there is provision for dynamic locking. Multiple end caps provide optimal length adjustment.

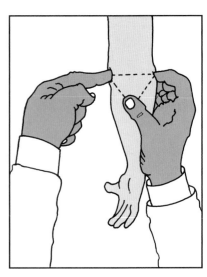

1. Definition: A supracondylar fracture of the humerus is a fracture which occurs in the distal third of the bone. The fracture line lies just proximal to the bone masses of the trochlea (1) and capitellum (capitulum) (2) and often runs through the apices of the coronoid (3) and olecranon fossae. The fracture line is generally transverse.

2. Occurrence: The supracondylar fracture is a common fracture of childhood; its incidence reaches a peak about the age of 8 years. It generally results from a fall on the outstretched hand, and should always be suspected when a child complains of pain in the elbow after such an injury.

3. Diagnosis: The olecranon and medial and lateral epicondyles preserve their normal equilateral triangular relationship (unlike dislocation of the elbow, also common in children). There is tenderness over the distal humerus, there may be marked swelling and deformity, and the child generally resists examination. Radiography is mandatory, but interpretation requires care.

4. Radiographs (a): Interpretation of radiographs of the elbow in children is made difficult by the changes produced by the successive appearance of ossification in the epiphyses. The old mnemonic 'cite' (capitellum, internal epicondyle, trochlea, ext. epicondyle) for appearance of the epiphyseal centres at 3, 6, 9 and 12 years is sufficiently accurate for normal purposes, but note that the capitulum may appear as early as the end of the first year.

5. Radiographs (b): Variations in appearances occur, and if there is any difficulty in interpreting the radiographs, there should be no hesitation in having films taken of the other side for direct comparison. These may for example draw attention to (1) the slight cortical irregularity of a minor greenstick fracture.

6. Radiographs (c): In fractures associated with more violence, the next detectable sign may be a hairline crack, visible in the AP view only (2). With more violence, the fracture line will be detectable in the lateral projection as well (3). Next, the distal fragment is tilted in a backward direction (4).

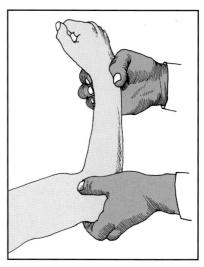

7. Radiographs (d): With still greater violence there is backward displacement (5), often leading to loss of bony contact. In the AP view there is often medial or lateral shift of the epiphyseal complex (M). The complex may also be rotated relative to the humeral shaft (generally lateral rotation). Rarely, as a result of other mechanisms the distal fragment is displaced and tilted anteriorly (A). Occult fractures may be suggested by the posterior fat pad becoming apparent in the lateral projections.

8. Vascular complications (a): Where there is appreciable displacement of the fracture, the brachial artery may be affected by the proximal fragment. In the majority of cases this is no more than a kinking of the vessel, but occasionally structural damage to the wall may occur, with the risk of Volkmann's ischaemic contracture. (Rarely the neurovascular bundle is trapped between the fracture and the biceps tendon, with tethering of the overlying skin; this is an indication for exploration.)

9. Vascular complications (b): In every case check and record the circulation prior to any manipulation. Seek the radial pulse, and note any evidence of arterial obstruction (pallor and coldness of the limb, pain and paraesthesia in the forearm, and progressive weakness of the forearm muscles). Look for excessive swelling and bruising round the elbow. **Neurological complications:** Note any evidence of impaired function in the ulnar, median or radial nerves, said to occur in 6–16% of cases.

10. Interpretation of radiographs (a): Certain *displacements* showing in the lateral give a clear guide to the necessity for reduction.
(1) Displacement with accompanying evidence of arterial obstruction. (This absolute also applies to angled fractures with vascular complications.)
(2) Displacements with complete loss of bony contact.
(3) Ideally, where the displacement is such that there is less than 50% of bony contact.

11. Interpretation of radiographs (b): (4) If there is *backward tilting* (anterior angulation) of the distal fragment by 15° or more, then correction should be attempted. Note that in the normal elbow the articular surfaces of the distal humerus lie at 45° to the axis of the humerus. (The construction is shown and the actual deformity is 20° (45-25°).) Remodelling of persistent angulation is slow and may be poor, leading to loss of flexion.

12. Interpretation of radiographs (c): (5) Reduction is required if there is significant *lateral or medial tilting*. Note that the normal 'carrying angle' of the elbow is about 10°. (Illustrated is a cubitus varus deformity of 17° (10 + 7°). Cubitus varus and cubitus valgus do not remodel well, and may ultimately be associated with tardy ulnar nerve palsy. Some regard any degree of tilting as significant and meriting correction, and certainly a deformity of 10° and above is unacceptable.

13. Interpretation of radiographs (d): (6)
Reduction is required if there is any significant *rotational* deformity. This is generally most obvious in the lateral projection. (Left above: no rotational (torsional) deformity present; Right: rotational deformity present.) Rotation, like cubitus valgus and varus, does not remodel well. In this context 'significant' is in effect any degree of rotation that is obvious in the plain films.

14. Classification of supracondylar fractures: Simple and useful is the Wilkins modification of the Gartland system: **Type I:** Undisplaced fracture; **Type IIa:** Greenstick fracture with anterior angulation (posterior tilting of the distal fragment); **Type IIb:** Greenstick fracture with anterior angulation and rotation; **Type III:** Completely displaced fracture. Types I and IIa do well, almost irrespective of treatment. *Results are poorer in Type IIb and Type III, and internal fixation is preferred by many for injuries in these categories.*

15. Summary of indications for reduction: Assuming no vascular complication, pure posterior displacement (1), lateral or medial displacement (2) of 50% or less, and angulation of less than 15° (3) *may be accepted, as remodelling is generally rapid and effective.* Rotation (4), valgus or varus (5), or loss of bony contact (6) require correction. In the next frames the techniques for closed reduction and cast fixation for any supracondylar fracture are followed by alternative methods using internal fixation.

16. Manipulation techniques (a): The arm should be manipulated under general anaesthesia. Gentle/moderate traction is applied at about 20° of flexion while an assistant applies counter-traction. This leads to disimpaction of the fracture. Some surgeons advise that this and the following stages should be carried out with the arm in supination.

17. Manipulation (b): Now maintaining traction and counter-traction (1) flex the elbow to 80° (2). This lifts the distal fragment, thereby reducing any posterior displacement and correcting any backward tilting (anterior angulation).

18. Manipulation (c): During this manoeuvre, the epiphyseal complex may be further coaxed into position by grasping it in the free hand. The thumb can be used to steady the proximal humeral shaft. Lateral displacement and torsional deformity (axial rotation) may also be corrected in this way.

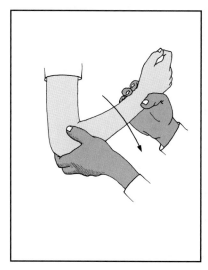

19. Fixation (a): After reduction, the fracture must be maintained in a stable position. Flexion of the elbow stretches the triceps over the fracture, often splinting it most efficiently. *The aim should be to flex the elbow as far as the state of the circulation at the time will permit, while making an allowance in anticipation of further swelling.*

20. Fixation (b): Assuming that at 80° a pulse is present (if present before the manipulation it should still be there, and if first absent it will have hopefully been restored) continue flexion of the elbow until the pulse disappears (due to the elbow flexure crease along with the swelling compressing the brachial artery).

21. Fixation (c): Now extend the elbow slowly for about 10° beyond the point when the pulse returns. *This is the position in which the arm should be maintained.* If 110–20° or more of flexion can be preserved, a sling and body bandage, well secured with adhesive strapping, may suffice for fixation.

22. Fixation (d): Unfortunately further extension of the elbow may be required to restore the circulation. In such cases, apply a generous layer of wool (1), followed by a long arm plaster slab (2) secured with bandages and a sling (3). *Many surgeons favour this in every case. **Warning:** never apply a complete* plaster because of the risks of swelling, and avoid applying any pressure with encircling bandages at the front of the elbow – some skirt this area, only bandaging the cast into position above and below the joint.

23. Fixation (e): While the slab is being applied, the risks of recurrence of valgus or varus deformity may be reduced by careful positioning of the forearm: viz. if there has been valgus deformity (lateral tilting, medical angulation) (1) place the arm in supination. With varus (2) Place the arm in pronation. With insignificant angulation the neutral position may be employed.

24. Check radiographs: Check radiographs must now be taken in two planes. (For interpretation of AP radiographs, see later.) In the lateral projection illustrated there has been a good reduction: note how all posterior displacement has been corrected and the normal angulation of the epiphyseal complex has been largely restored. (For key see following frame.)

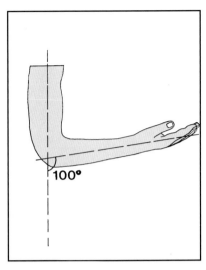

25. Check lateral radiographs *ctd:* This diagram is based on the previous radiograph, and shows correction of all posterior displacement (1), and restoration of the normal angulation of the epiphyseal complex (2). (F = fracture line; C = capitellum; R = radial head.) If a good reduction has been achieved:
1. discontinue the anaesthetic; 2. admit the child for overnight observation; 3. elevate the arm in a roller towel or similar device; 4. leave access in the dressings for observation of the pulse and finger circulation.

26. Late development of ischaemia: If while under observation the pulse disappears, and especially if there are other signs of ischaemia, *all* encircling bandages should be cut, and *all* wool in front of the elbow teased out. If this does not lead to improvement, the elbow should be placed in a more extended position (e.g. by cracking the slab and slackening the sling).

27. Absent pulse after manipulation: Returning to Frame 20: If after manipulation the pulse is *not* palpable, the elbow should be flexed to *not more than 100°* and maintained in that position with a sling and a back slab (applied over wool and held with a lightly applied bandage). The anaesthetic should be continued while check radiographs are taken.

28. Radiographs (a): If the radiographs show a poor reduction, then no more than two further attempts at manipulation may be permitted under the same anaesthetic. The illustration shows a typical unsatisfactory lateral projection where there is complete loss of contact between the distal fragment and the humeral shaft, with proximal displacement of the distal fragment (compare with Frame 24).

29. Radiographs (b): an AP projection should also be taken and the position checked in every case, even although faults in reduction demonstrated in the lateral projection are the ones more usually associated with circulatory impairment. As the AP view cannot be obtained with the elbow straight, superimposition of the radius, ulna and humerus make interpretation difficult (but see following frame). Be careful to avoid disturbing the reduction during the taking of these radiographs.

30. Radiographs (c): The epiphyseal complex preserves its relationship with the radius and ulna. In turn, with a good reduction, the radius and ulna regain their alignment with the humerus. Note in this unsatisfactory reduction the radius (R), ulna (U) and epiphyseal complex (E) are displaced medially in relationship to the humerus (H).

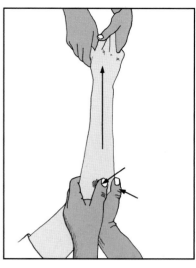

31. Radiographs (d): The preceding case with vascular impairment was remanipulated and the above correction obtained. This is a good reduction, and was accompanied by restoration of the pulse at the wrist.

32. Radiographs (e): A line drawing of the preceding radiograph is shown along with a sketch of the forearm bones drawn in roughly the same position (compare also with Frame 29). (R) = radius, (U) = ulna, (H) = humerus, (F) = fracture, (O) = olecranon, (M) = medial epicondyle.

33. Remanipulation: If a poor reduction has been obtained and remanipulation is necessary, the preceding technique may be repeated; alternatively, while an assistant applies light traction to the forearm, the distal fragment is pushed forwards with the thumb while the fingers control the proximal fragment. Plaster fixation may be applied as described before.

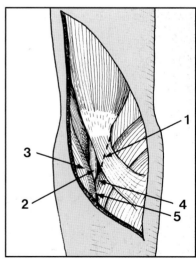

34. Absent pulse, adequate circulation: If a good reduction has been obtained and the pulse remains absent (this occurs in 3% of cases) the circulation should be checked more critically. The use of a pulse oximeter before and after manipulation is often helpful. If the hand is warm and pink, with good capillary return in the nails, there is no immediate indication for further intervention. *Admission, elevation and close observation for 24 hours* are essential. (Generally the pulse returns spontaneously over 2–3 days.)

35. Absent pulse, ischaemia: If there are incontrovertible signs of gross ischaemia, either in the face of a good reduction or a failed reduction, *exploration of the brachial artery* must now be undertaken. (Volkmann's ischaemic contracture occurs roughly once in every thousand cases of supracondylar fracture, and is generally avoidable.) Exposure of the artery is straightforward. (i) A lazy S incision may be used, following the lateral edge of biceps and crossing the elbow near the fold.

36. Exploration of brachial artery *ctd:* (ii) The skin edges are reflected and the bicipital aponeurosis (1) divided close to the tendon (iii) The arm is put in full pronation and the space (5) between brachioradialis laterally (3) and pronator teres medially (4) opened up with the finger tips.

37. Exploration brachial artery *ctd:* (iv) The brachial artery (A) is found lying close to the biceps tendon. The median nerve (M) lies on its medial side. The fracture lies deep to the brachialis (B) in the floor of the wound. In some cases relief of local pressure on the vessel (e.g. from the fracture) may restore the circulation, but other measures, requiring experience in vascular surgery, may be necessary.

38. Reduction failure with satisfactory circulation (a): it is unwise to repeat manipulation beyond the third attempt owing to the risks of increasing swelling. In these circumstances, marked displacement (but not angulation, valgus or varus) may be accepted, relying on later remodelling. The fracture illustrated had no bony contact (completely off-ended) in the lateral: after a year, considerable remodelling has occurred, with loss of 15° only of flexion.

39. Reduction failure (b): If displacement and angulation are outside acceptable limits, open reduction is not generally recommended. Instead, continuous traction may be employed. This is especially indicated where there is minimal circulatory impairment, brachial artery exploration is not indicated, and the elbow cannot be flexed. In *Dunlop traction,* traction tapes are applied to the limb. (W) = wool; (C) = lightly applied crepe bandage.

40. Reduction failure (c): The arm is abducted at the shoulder and traction of 1.5 kg applied with the elbow at 60° flexion. Counter-traction of 1 kg is applied directly with a canvas sling applied well above the elbow to avoid compression in this vulnerable area. After swelling subsides the situation may be re-appraised, or the traction discontinued and a plaster slab substituted at 2–3 weeks.

41. Reduction failure (d): As an alternative to Dunlop traction (and also as a routine treatment) Gadgil et al[1] recommend straight arm traction with the arm in 90° abduction and the shoulder elevated from the bed, using skin tapes applied under opiate analgesia. Minor adjustments allow good control of any tendency to cubitus varus or valgus. Weekly radiographs are taken, and traction stopped when the patient can actively flex the elbow. The best results were obtained in children under 10 years, and a disadvantage is the time in hospital.

42. Reduction failure (e): Alternatively skeletal traction may be employed: this may be achieved with a butterfly (wing) screw or similar device in the ulna. Traction is applied with weights, and the forearm supported by a sling. Elbow flexion may be controlled with the sling which may be elevated or lowered as thought necessary: this avoids any direct pressure in the antecubital fossa.

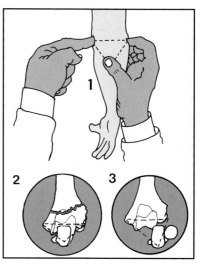

79. Intercondylar fractures (c): In displaced and moderately fragmented fractures, especially in the younger patient, open reduction should be carried out. *Approaches:* (a) through a lateral incision (b) through a triceps splitting incision, or (c) through a chevron osteotomy of the olecranon (1) with its proximal reflection (triceps attached) (2). *Reduction*: The articular fragments should be reduced first using Kirschner wires: it may be helpful to manipulate the lateral element using a wire inserted in the retrograde fashion (a, b, c).

80. Intercondylar fractures (d): After reduction there is a wide choice of internal fixation devices which may be used to secure the position of the fragments. Common methods include the following: (a) = LCP Distal Humeral Plates; (b) = Locking Compression Plates; (c) = Zimmer Pre-Contoured Periarticular Plates. The aim should be to obtain fixation which is robust enough to permit early mobilisation of the joint.

81. Dislocation of the elbow (a): Dislocation of the elbow is common in both children and adults and generally results from a fall on the outstretched hand. It is sometimes confused with a supracondylar fracture. The two may be distinguished clinically by searching for the equilateral triangle formed by the olecranon and epicondyles (1). This is undisturbed in supracondylar fractures (2) but distorted in elbow dislocations (3).

82. Dislocation of the elbow (b): Damage to the ulnar nerve, median nerve or brachial artery is uncommon, but nevertheless should always be sought. A number of motor tests may be used to assess function in both nerves. *In the case of the ulnar nerve* the ability to grip a sheet of paper between the ring and little finger (1) may be used to assess good interosseous muscle function. It is important that the fingers are not allowed to flex at the MP joints. *In the case of the median nerve* contraction and power in abductor pollicis may be assessed by feeling the muscle (2) while the patient attempts to resist the thumb being pressed from a vertical position into the plane of the palm. Sensory function in the areas supplied by the median and ulnar nerves should also be quickly tested (3). *In the case of the brachial artery* the quickest assessment is of course by identification of the radial pulse (4).

83. Radiographs: The radiograph above shows the typical appearances in the AP projection of a dislocation of the elbow. Note how the radius and ulna are displaced laterally and proximally.

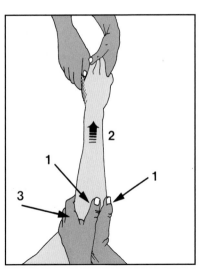

84. Radiographs *ctd:* The lateral shows posterior and proximal displacement. These combined appearances are those found in the commonest dislocation of the elbow, the posterolateral dislocation. Accompanying fractures are uncommon, but it is a wise to assume that there is an associated injury until you have demonstrated otherwise.
In particular, post reduction films should be carefully scrutinised. In adults, look for fractures of the coronoid process and the radial head, and in children, the epicondyles or the lateral condyle.

85. Treatment (a): Reduction should be carried out under general anaesthesia. A fair amount of force is often required, although the use of a muscle relaxant will reduce this. Apply strong traction in the line of the limb, and if necessary slightly flex the elbow while maintaining traction. Success is usually accompanied with a characteristic reduction 'clunk'.

86. Treatment (b): If the last manoeuvre is unsuccessful, clasp the arm and push the olecranon forwards and medially (1), using traction in moderate flexion (2) and counter-traction with the fingers (3).

87. Treatment (c): After reduction has been achieved, take check radiographs, and apply a padded crepe bandage; this may be worn with a sling for 2 weeks (4). Alternatively, apply a plaster back slab and sling with the elbow in 90° flexion (5). Avoid too early or too vigorous mobilisation, and passive movements which run the risk of precipitating myositis ossificans.

88. Late diagnosed posterior dislocation in children: Between 3 weeks and 2 months, open reduction carries an unacceptable risk of myositis ossificans; if the dislocation is discovered within that period the injury should be treated conservatively and the elbow just mobilised. A quarter do well and need no further treatment; in the remainder (and in cases discovered later than two months) operative reduction should be attempted.

Late diagnosed posterior dislocation in adults: In the adult soft tissue contractures render manipulative reduction impossible. After their operative release it is generally the case that congruency of the articular surfaces can only be maintained by immobilisation. Unfortunately this is almost inevitably followed by stiffness which may cause considerable loss of function. In these circumstances good results have been claimed by performing a primary semi-constrained total elbow arthroplasty.[3]

89. Associated injuries (a): In children, the medial epicondylar epiphysis may be detached. *On reduction of the elbow,* it will generally be restored to an acceptable position. A plaster slab and a sling are advised for 4 weeks.
(b) *The medial epicondyle may be retained in the joint:* this must always be excluded (see Frame 55 et seq.).

90. Associated injuries (c): Lateral condylar injury: Note the following points. 1. The capitellar epiphysis (along with half the cartilaginous trochlea) has been carried medially by the radius, and is slightly rotated. 2. The medial epicondylar epiphysis has just appeared and is not displaced. 3. The *medial* dislocation of the elbow is unusual.

91. Associated injuries: Lateral condylar injuries *ctd:* The preceding injury was treated by manipulative reduction; the lateral condylar complex remained displaced. (Reduction could be achieved by firm local pressure, but displacement occurred in this unstable injury as soon as pressure was released.)

92. Associated injuries: Lateral condylar injuries *ctd:* Open reduction was therefore carried out and the condylar mass held in position with two Kirschner wires. Note the small bone fragment from the shaft (Salter/Harris Type 2 injury). Fixation was complemented by a long arm plaster back shell for 4 weeks.

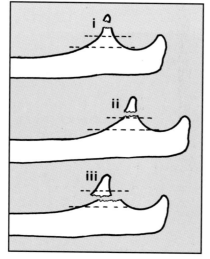

93. Associated injuries in the adult: the terrible triad (a): This name is given to a dislocation of the elbow with associated fractures of the radial head and the coronoid. Complications are common and the clinical outcome usually poor. The combination of fracture and collateral ligament damage may lead to instability, delayed mobilisation, and elbow stiffness. (Illus. Posterior dislocation of the elbow with a Type 3 fracture of the radial head (see p. 171)).

94. Associated injuries in the adult: the terrible triad (b): Coronoid fractures associated with elbow dislocations (and those occurring on their own) can be classified into three grades: Grade 1, simple avulsions (i); Grade 2, fractures involving half or less of the coronoid (ii); Grade 3, fractures involving more than half (iii).

Treatment protocols
1. If the fractures are minimally displaced the elbow should be reduced by manipulation as previously described. Then, if the elbow is found to be stable in the range 30–130°, the injury should be treated conservatively.
2. Conservative treatment is also advised in patients who are medically unfit for a prolonged procedure, or if they are non-compliant.
3. *In all others surgical repair is considered to offer the best prospects for recovery.*[4]

Surgical treatment
1. After manipulative or open reduction the coronoid is fixed: if the fragment is substantial (Grade 2 or 3) it may be held with a screw. If small (Grade 1), it may be held in a reduced position by using a lasso suture passed through holes drilled in the base of the coronoid.
2. If possible the radial head should be reduced and the fragments held with small screws or an appropriate plate and screws. If the degree of comminution precludes this, the fragments should be carefully removed and a metal (rather than silastic) head replacement carried out.
3. The lateral ligament complex should be repaired.
4. Where there is remaining instability the medial collateral ligament complex should be repaired and /or a hinged external fixator applied.

(Isolated fractures of the coronoid, if associated with instability should be treated as indicated above.)

95. Anterior dislocation of the elbow (a): This is an uncommon injury, but may follow a fall on the elbow which results in the forearm bones being pushed forwards. For dislocation to occur, the olecranon must fracture, and this becomes a potentially very unstable injury (see also Chapter 8, p. 186).

96. Anterior dislocation (b): The elbow may be reduced by applying traction and extending the joint. If the reduction is stable, it may then be treated by plaster fixation for a limited period in extension as in an anterior supracondylar fracture. Nevertheless, there is appreciable risk of late subluxation and difficulty in elbow mobilisation so that, on the whole, internal fixation is recommended for this injury (Illus: a Rush pin with tension band wiring: see Frame 98 for a preferred position for the wire).

97. Anterior dislocation (c): A more complex form of anterior dislocation is seen in the side swipe injury ('baby car fracture'). This occurs when a driver rests his elbow on his car's window ledge, and he is struck by a passing vehicle. Typically the elements of this injury include (1) anterior dislocation of the elbow with fractures of (2) the olecranon (3), the humerus (4), the ulna and sometimes (5) the radius.

98. Anterior dislocation (d): It is vital to reduce and hold the dislocation immediately; thereafter the accompanying injuries should be fixed if at all possible at the same sitting. (Illus: olecranon fracture held with a screw and tension band wiring; ulnar fracture held with intramedullary device (Rush pin); ideally the humeral fracture would also be internally fixed.) If damage control orthopaedics will not permit such a lengthy procedure, reduce the dislocation, and keep the elbow in extension in a cast for 2–3 weeks prior to delayed internal fixation.

99. Isolated dislocation of the ulna: Dislocation of the ulna may occur in association with a fracture of the radial shaft. As such fractures may be quite distal, it is important that adequate radiographs of the forearm are taken. This double injury may be treated by manipulative reduction of the elbow followed by a long arm plaster until the radius has united. However, to permit early mobilisation and the avoidance of elbow stiffness, internal fixation of the radius is to be preferred.

100. Isolated dislocation of the radius: Lateral, anterior or posterior dislocation of the proximal end of the radius is almost invariably part of a Monteggia lesion (see p. 186) which is sometimes concealed because the ulnar fracture is of greenstick pattern (Illus.). Great care must be taken in the assessment and treatment of these injuries which is dealt with in detail later. (See pp 186–188.)

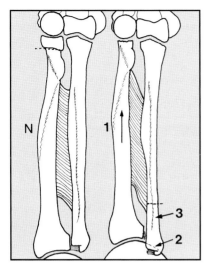

124. Treatment (g): Sometimes excision is followed with pain and weakness, cubitus valgus, and osteoarthritis. There may also be proximal drift of the radius (1) so that the distal end of the ulna becomes prominent and painful (2). This may be treated by excision of the distal end of the ulna, albeit with some weakening of the grip. Proximal drift is a feature of the Essex–Lopresti lesion, and may be minimised by delaying radial head excision for 6 weeks.

125. Fractures of the radial neck (a): The axis of rotation of the radio-ulnar joints passes through the centre of the radial head (1) and the attachment of the triangular fibrocartilage (2). The axis passes through the centre of the neck (3) and lies at right angles to the plane of the head. Fractures through the neck (4) have the potential to disturb this relationship between the head and the neck.

126. Fractures of the radial neck (b): Fractures of the radial neck may result from the same mechanisms as those causing fractures of the radial head, and the diagnostic features are also similar. Patterns: The fractures may be hair-line and undisplaced (1) or result in slight (2) or gross tilting (3). In children, the epiphysis of the head may be completely separated and widely displaced (4).

127. Treatment (a): With slight or no tilting (1 and 2) and up to 30° in children treat conservatively (as in Frame 118). With marked tilting (3) (20° or more in adults) manipulate. Do so by applying traction and gently pronate and supinate, feeling for the prominent part of the radial head to present; then apply pressure when the head is at its zenith. (Thereafter treat as in frame 118.) Open reduction is indicated if closed methods fail.

128. Treatment (b): Where there is gross epiphyseal displacement, operative reduction is indicated. On reduction, the fragments may be found to lock in a stable position. If not, a Kirschner wire may be used for 2–3 weeks to achieve stability. *Note*: In some cases of severe tilting it is possible to obtain a reduction by inserting a temporary percutaneous wire into the radial head and levering it back into position under intensifier control.

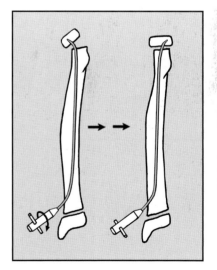

129. Treatment (c): As an alternative, Prathapkumar et al[5] claim good results using a Nancy nail. One with a sharp tip is bent to 45° (in order to capture the displaced epiphysis). It is then inserted 2 cm proximal to the distal radial epiphysis under general anaesthesia and intensifier control. Once a good hold has been obtained in the epiphysis, rotation of the nail (the direction being dependent on the displacement), along with local pressure, leads to reduction. The distal end is then trimmed to within 1 cm of the bone.

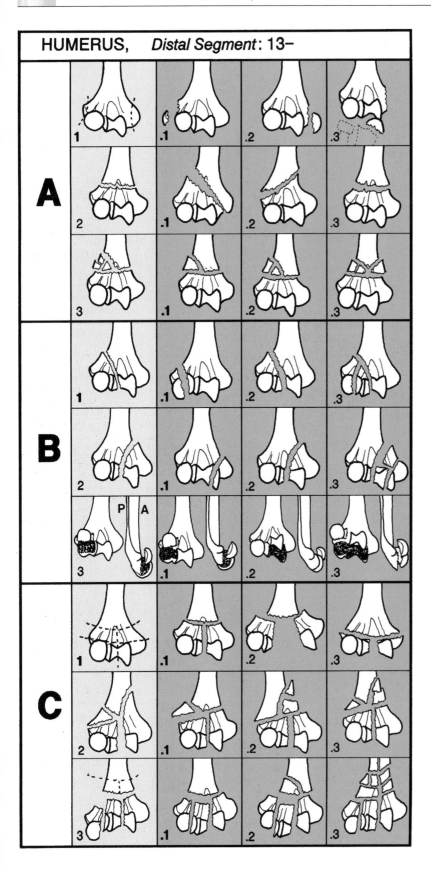

HUMERUS, *Distal Segment*: 13–

130. AO Classification of fractures of the humerus, distal segment (13–):

Type A fractures are totally extra-articular.
A1 = Avulsion fracture (of apophysis):
.1 lateral; .2 medial; .3 medial, with the fragment trapped in the joint.
A2 = Simple metaphyseal (supracondylar fracture): .1 with the proximal part of the fracture line lying lateral; .2 with proximal part of the fracture line lying medial; .3 with the fracture line lying transverse.
A3 = Multifragmented metaphyseal;
.1 with an unbroken wedge; .2 with the wedge fragment fractured; .3 complex.

Type B fractures are partially articular.
B1 = Lateral sagittal (i.e. generally most obvious in the AP radiographic projection):
.1 involving the capitellum; .2 simple trochlear; .3 multifragmentary trochlear.
B2 = Medial sagittal: .1 medial side of the trochlea; .2 through the trochlear notch;
.3 multifragmentary trochlear.
B3 = Frontal (i.e. generally most obvious in the lateral radiographic projection): .1 of the capitellum; .2 of the trochlea; .3 of both the capitellum and the trochlea.

Type C fractures are complete articular fractures, and are multifragmentary.
C1 = Simple fractures of both the epiphysis and the metaphysis (T- and Y-fractures):
.1 slight displacement only; .2 with marked displacement; .3 T-fractures with the horizontal limb distally placed so that it is in the epiphysis.
C2 = Simple fracture of the epiphysis, multifragmentary fracture of the metaphysis: .1 wedge intact; .2 wedge fractured; .3 complex.
C3 = Multifragmentary epiphyseal fracture with a simple or multi fragmentary fracture of the metaphysis; .1 metaphysis simple;
.2 wedge fracture of the metaphysis;
.3 complex metaphyseal fracture.

8

Injuries to the forearm bones

Note:

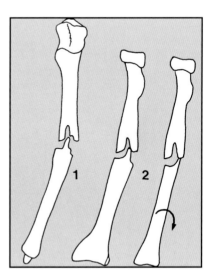

1. Anatomical features: The radius and ulna are bound together by (1) the annular (orbicular) ligament, (2) the interosseous membrane, (3) the radio-ulnar ligaments and the triangular fibrocartilage. This gives the radius and ulna some of the features of (4) a bundle of sticks and (5) a linked parallelogram.

2. Direct violence: With direct violence it is possible to fracture either of the forearm bones in isolation. These injuries are comparatively uncommon, but do occur, especially in the ulna when in a fall the shaft strikes a hard edge. They may also occur when the ulna is struck by a weapon as the victim attempts to protect his head with his arms.

3. Indirect violence: More commonly the forearm is injured as the result of indirect violence, such as a fall on the back or the front of the outstretched hand. The force of impact on the hand stresses the forearm bones: the most common occurrence is for both to fracture.

4. Fracture–dislocations (a): If *one* forearm bone is seen to be fractured and angled, it has inevitably become relatively shorter (1). If its attachments to the wrist and humerus are intact, the other forearm bone *must* be dislocated. The commonest fracture–dislocation of this type is a fracture of the ulna with a dislocation of the radial head (Monteggia injury) (2).

5. Fracture–dislocation (b): The same pattern of injury occurs in the Galeazzi fracture–dislocation when a dislocation of the distal ulna accompanies a shaft fracture of the radius. *Never accept a single forearm bone fracture as an entity until a Monteggia or Galeazzi injury has been eliminated.*

6. Axial rotation (a): In any forearm injury, when the ulna fractures it may angulate or displace like any other bone (1). When the radius fractures, however, *in addition* to angulation one fragment may rotate relative to the other (axial rotation) (2).

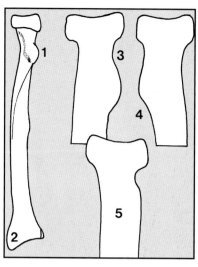

7. Axial rotation (b): Axial rotation of the ulna is rare, but always check to see that it is not present. To do so, note that in the lateral projection the olecranon (1), coronoid (2) and styloid process (3) should be clearly visible. This relationship is lost in the presence of axial rotation (4).

8. Axial rotation (c): In the case of the radius, note any discrepancy in the widths of the fragments at fracture level. A difference as illustrated indicates the presence of axial rotation.

9. Axial rotation (d): Note also the normal relationship between the radial tubercle (1) and the styloid process (2) in this AP view of the radius in full supination. In *full supination* the radial tubercle lies *medially* (3). In *pronation* it lies *laterally* (4). In the mid position it is concealed (5). The position of the radial styloid should always correspond.

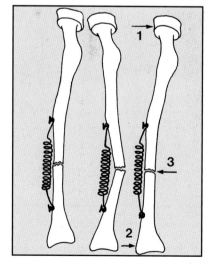

10. Axial rotation (e): Forces responsible (i): In all radial shaft fractures, pronator quadratus tends to pronate the distal fragment (1). In all upper (proximal) third fractures, pronator teres helps to pronate the distal fragment (2), assisting pronator quadratus in this movement.

11. Axial rotation (f): Forces responsible (ii): In upper third fractures, the proximal fragment is fully supinated by biceps (3) while the distal fragment is fully pronated by pronators teres and quadratus (1 and 2), (i.e. there is a maximal tendency to axial rotation). In fractures distal to the mid third, biceps is opposed, so the proximal fragment tends to lie in the mid position.

12. Fracture slipping (a): Greenstick fractures: In children's greenstick fractures any intact periosteum on the original concave surface of the fracture exerts a constant, springy force which may cause recurrence of angulation if the plaster slackens, impairing three-point fixation. *Frequent check films may be essential in any conservatively treated fracture.*

13. Fracture slipping (b): Another contributory cause of fracture slipping is when muscle wasting occurs in a patient in a full arm plaster wearing a collar and cuff sling. Loss of brachialis and brachioradialis bulk leads to plaster slackening and angulatory deformity. (*Note:* the soft tissue shadows in Frame 29) *Patients with conservatively treated fractures should be given broad arm slings.*

14. Fracture of both bones of the forearm in children: Patterns (a): Most fractures are greenstick in pattern as illustrated. The radiograph shows fractures of the radius and ulna in the middle thirds. The distal fragments are tilted anteriorly (posterior angulation) but there is no displacement. An extensive, intact periosteal hinge can be assumed and reduction of such a fracture involves correction of the angulation only.

15. Patterns (b): When there is off-ending of one or both bones there is potential instability. Shortening and angulation are more likely, and axial rotation may occur; reduction and the maintenance of reduction may therefore be more troublesome.

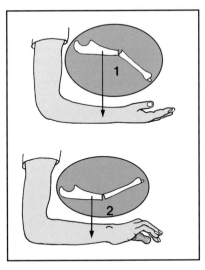

16. Treatment (a): In the undisplaced angulated greenstick fracture, the child should be given a general anaesthetic and the angulation corrected. One hand applies a little traction and the corrective force, while the other acts as a fulcrum, under the fracture.

17. Treatment (b): If the fracture is overcorrected, the periosteum on the initially concave side of the fracture will be felt to snap. This will immediately give the fracture more mobility: this has the advantage of reducing the risks of late angulation, but has the disadvantage of requiring greater care with respect to the initial positioning in plaster.

18. Treatment (c): In the undisplaced greenstick fracture where there is no rotational deformity, the arm should be placed in a stable position while the cast is applied. To prevent re-angulation, *fractures with posterior tilting* (anterior angulation) (1) are generally most stable in full pronation, while *the commonest fractures with anterior tilting* (posterior angulation) (2) are best in full supination. If an extreme position is required, the cast should be changed at 4 weeks and the arm put in a more neutral position.

54. Galeazzi fracture: Treatment (b): If displacement of the ulna persists after internal fixation of the radius, a K-wire for 3 weeks may be used to stabilise the inferior radio-ulnar joint.
Galeazzi fracture–dislocations in children: Manipulate and put up in plaster in supination. Open reduction is seldom required.
Late diagnosed Galeazzi lesions: Prominence of the ulna with pain in the wrist is the commonest complaint and excision of the distal ulna may give relief.

55. Isolated fracture of the radius (a): Fracture of the radius can occur without initial involvement of the inferior radio-ulnar joint. This comparatively uncommon situation may follow direct injury to the radius which results in an undisplaced fracture. Nevertheless, late subluxation of the inferior radio-ulnar joint may appear when, as is frequent, late angulation of the fracture occurs.

56. Isolated fracture of the radius (b): *In the adult,* isolated fractures of the radius with no significant angulation or rotational deformity may be treated in plaster with the arm in supination. Slight axial rotation may be controlled by careful positioning of the forearm; in all cases careful surveillance is vital to detect early slipping, an indication for operative intervention.

In children, isolated fractures of the radius should also be treated conservatively.

Non-union of the radius: This complication may be treated along standard lines by internal fixation and bone grafting.

57. Forearm compartment syndromes: These occur most frequently after fractures of both the forearm bones, but may follow supracondylar fractures and fractures of the radial head and neck in children. The condition should be suspected if 1. there is marked pain, exacerbated by passive extension of the fingers; 2. there is reduced sensation or paraesthesia in the hand; 3. if there is a significant rise in compartment pressure: this is most useful in the unconscious patient.
Both anterior and posterior compartments may be affected, but the anterior is most commonly involved. (Release of pressure in the anterior compartment usually results in a fall of pressure in the posterior compartment: but if pressure monitoring shows pressure in the posterior compartment separate decompression (through a separate, linear posterior incision) may be required.

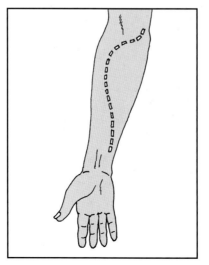

Method: A curvilinear incision is generally advised. (McConnell's approach (Illus.) as described by Henry not only allows decompression of the anterior compartment, but exposure (if required) of both the median and ulnar nerves.) The decompression must include:
(a) the lacertus fibrosus (bicipital aponeurosis)
(b) the fascia over flexor carpi ulnaris
(c) the fascia over the edge of flexor digitorum superficialis.

If injury to the median nerve is suspected, the likely sites of its compression are:
(a) at the lacertus
(b) over the proximal margin of pronator teres
(c) at the proximal margin of flexor digitorum superficialis.

RADIUS/ULNA, *Diaphyseal Segment* : 22–

58. AO Classification of fractures of the radius/ulna, diaphyseal segment (22–):

Type A are simple (i.e. there is a circumferential disruption of the bone), involving one or both bones.
A1 = Simple fracture of the ulna with an intact radius: .1 oblique; .2 transverse; .3 with dislocation of the radial head (Monteggia fracture–dislocation).
A2 = Simple fracture of the radius, with the ulna intact: .1 oblique; .2 transverse; .3 with dislocation of the distal radio-ulnar joint (Galeazzi fracture–dislocation).
A3 = Simple fracture of both bones: .1 proximal part of radius involved; .2 middle third of radius fractured; .3 fracture of distal radius.

Type B fractures are wedge fractures (i.e. there is a separate (butterfly) segment, but after reduction there is contact between the main fragments (a so-called hitch)); one or both bones are involved.
B1 = Wedge fracture of the ulna and an intact radius; .1 wedge intact; .2 multifragmentary wedge; .3 with dislocation of the radial head (Monteggia fracture–dislocation).
B2 = Wedge fracture of the radius and an intact ulna: .1 wedge intact;
.2 multifragmentary wedge;
.3 with dislocation of the distal radio-ulnar joint (Galeazzi fracture–dislocation).
B3 = Wedge fracture of one bone, with a simple or wedge fracture of the other: .1 wedge ulna; .2 wedge radius; .3 wedge fractures of both bones.

Type C fractures are complex (i.e. they have more than two fragments, and even after reduction the pattern is such that there is no contact between the main fragments); one or both bones may be involved.
C1 = Complex fracture of the ulna: .1 bifocal with an intact radius; .2 bifocal, with the radius fractured; .3 irregular, with or without fracture of the radius.
C2 = Complex fracture of the radius:
.1 bifocal ulna intact; .2 bifocal with a fracture of the ulna; .3 irregular, with or without a fracture of the ulna.
C3 = Complex fracture of both bones; .1 bifocal of both bones; .2 bifocal of one bone and irregular fracture of the other; .3 irregular fracture of both bones.

19. Reduction technique (b): Before any manipulation, start by preparing a suitable plaster back slab. The *length* should equal the distance from the olecranon to the metacarpal heads (1). The *width* in an adult should be 15 cm (6″), and it should be about eight layers thick. The slab should be trimmed with a tongue (2) for the first web space, a large radial curve to allow elbow flexion (3) and allowance for ulnar deviation (4).

20. Reduction technique (c): The essential first stage in the reduction of a Colles fracture is to disimpact the distal radial fragment. The elbow is flexed to a right angle and the arm held by the interlocked fingers of an assistant (1). Traction is applied in the line of the forearm (2).

21. Reduction technique (d): Traction need only be applied for a few seconds, and disimpaction may be confirmed by holding the distal fragment between the thumb and index. It should be easy to move anteriorly and posteriorly. When disimpacted the radial styloid should lie 1 cm distal to the ulnar styloid.

22. Reduction technique (e): The elbow is now extended (1). The heel of one hand should be placed over the dorsal surface of the distal radial fragment, and the fingers curled round the patient's wrist and palm (2). This grip allows traction to be re-applied to the disimpacted fracture.

23. Reduction technique (f): Now, by using the heel of the other hand as a fulcrum (3) firm pressure directed anteriorly (4) will correct all the remaining deformities normally visible in lateral radiographs of the wrist (posterior displacement, anterior angulation).

24. Reduction technique (g): Still maintaining traction, alter the position of the grip so that the heel (here of the right hand) is able to push the distal fragment ulnarwards and correct the radial displacement (5). Ulnar angulation, the other deformity seen in the AP radiograph, is corrected by placing the hand in full ulnar deviation at the wrist.

25. Reduction technique (h): Change the grip to allow free application of the plaster (which follows Charnley's principle of three point fixation). Note that one hand holds the thumb fully extended (1). The other holds three fingers (to avoid 'cupping' of the hand) maintaining slight traction (2). The limb should be in full pronation (3), *full* ulnar deviation at the wrist (4) and *slight* palmar flexion.

26. Reduction technique (i): Note that the elbow must be *extended* (either by an assistant (5) or by resting the upper arm against the edge of the table) to maintain this position. The skin may be protected with wool roll (6). If stockingette is preferred, it must be applied prior to reduction.

27. Reduction technique (j): The wetted slab should now be positioned so that it covers the anterior, lateral and posterior aspects of the radius (7). The tongue should be carefully turned into the palm (8). The slab should be held in position with two wetted 10 cm (4″) open-weave bandages (cotton, gauze or Kling™ bandages) (9). The end can be secured with a wetted scrap of plaster bandage.

28. Reduction technique (k): Before the plaster sets, many surgeons like to apply further pressure over the posterolateral aspect of the distal fragment, and maintain this until setting occurs ('final moulding'). This precaution ensures maintenance of the reduction, but care should be taken not to dent the plaster.

29. Reduction technique (l): A collar and cuff sling should be applied (1). Make sure that there is no constriction at the elbow (2) or at the wrist (3), and try to flex the elbow beyond a right angle so that the forearm is not dependent.

30. Alternative techniques: It is not unexpected that in this common fracture methods of reduction are legion. As it is generally an easy fracture to reduce, it follows that success can rightly be claimed for many techniques. The method given is logical in so far as it correlates with the pathology as seen on the radiographs.

Note, however:

(a) A direct, simple and extremely effective procedure is to disimpact the fracture (Frame 20), apply a plaster slab (Frame 27) and correct the deformity before the plaster sets by applying pressure on the posterolateral aspect of the distal fragment (as in Frame 28).

(b) In the elderly patient, unfit for general anaesthesia (but preferably after intravenous diazepam) a *marked* dorsal displacement may be corrected by quick application of pressure (without previous disimpaction) over a dorsal slab.

(c) In the young adult, if a good reduction cannot be secured and held, so that there is recurrence of severe deformity, the use of an external fixator, Kirschner wires or plating should be considered (see Frame 43 et seq).

24 hrs

2 – 5 days

31. Treatment *ctd:* Check radiographs should be studied. Severe persisting deformity, *especially in the AP projection* (Illus.) should not be accepted, and remanipulation should be undertaken. If difficulty is anticipated, radiographs may be obtained before discontinuing the anaesthetic. If the position is acceptable, the patient is shown finger exercises and advised regarding normal plaster care.

32. Aftercare (a): The patient is seen the next day and the fingers examined for adequacy of the circulation and the degree of swelling (1). The palm, fingers, thumb and elbow are checked for constriction caused by bandaging or elbow flexion, and any adjustments made (2). Thereafter the patient should be seen within the next 2-5 days with a view to completion of the plaster.

33. Aftercare (b): At the next review (usually a fracture clinic) finger swelling is checked: if slight, the plaster is completed (if marked, completion is delayed). *Superficial* layers of cotton bandage are removed, the slab retained, and encircling plaster bandages applied. The patient is instructed in elbow and shoulder exercises, and unless there is still a fair amount of swelling the sling may be discarded.

2/52

34. Aftercare (c): At 2 weeks the plaster is checked for marked slackening (replace), softening (reinforce) and technical faults (see next two frames). Movements in the fingers, elbow and shoulder are examined and appropriate advice given or physiotherapy started. In some centres radiographs are taken at this stage; slight slipping is inevitable, but marked slipping may be an indication for remanipulation (not usually a profitable procedure). At this stage too, if desired, the plaster may be replaced by a resin cast.

35. Aftercare (d): Positional errors: (1) The commonest fault is lack of ulnar deviation. This should be sadly accepted if discovered at 2 weeks (but replastered in the correct position if discovered earlier). Lack of ulnar deviation increases the risks of late problems arising from disruption of the inferior radio-ulnar joint; non-union of the ulnar styloid is common, with frequently some restriction of pronation and supination and local pain. (2) Excessive wrist flexion is liable to lead to difficulty in recovering dorsiflexion and a useful grip, and may be associated with compression of the median nerve. If present, the plaster should be re-applied with the wrist in a more extended position. (Full wrist flexion was once advocated in the treatment of Colles fracture - the Cotton-Loder position - but has been abandoned for the reasons given.)

36. Aftercare (e): Plaster faults: Errors in plastering technique should not occur, but nevertheless are often discovered at this stage. The following faults are common: (1) The distal edge of the plaster does not follow the normal oblique line of the MP joints, and movements of the little and sometimes the ring finger are restricted. The plaster should be trimmed to the dotted line. (2) All the MP joints are restricted by the plaster which has been continued beyond the palmar crease. Trim to the dotted line. (3) The thumb is restricted by a few turns of plaster bandage. Again the plaster should be trimmed to permit free movement. (4) The plaster is digging into the skin of the first web and should be trimmed back to the dotted line. (5) The plaster is too short. Support of the fracture is greatly impaired; the plaster should be extended to the olecranon behind, and as far in front as will still permit elbow flexion.

37. Aftercare (f): The plaster should be removed at 5 weeks (or 6 weeks in badly displaced fractures in the elderly) and the fracture assessed for union. (Radiographs are of limited value.) *If there is marked persisting tenderness*, a fresh plaster should be applied and union re-assessed in a further 2 weeks.

38. Aftercare (g): If tenderness is minimal or absent, (1) a circular woven support (e.g. Tubigrip™ or a crepe bandage) may be applied to limit oedema and to some extent increase the patient's confidence. (2) The patient is instructed in wrist and finger exercises and encouraged to practise these frequently and with vigour. Arrangements are made to review the patient in a further 2 weeks.

39. Need for rehabilitation (a): At about 7 weeks post injury, you must decide whether to discharge the patient or refer her for rehabilitation. Base your decision on: (i) finger movements, (ii) grip strength, (iii) wrist movements, (iv) the patient's occupation. For example, 1. if finger 'tuck-in' (i.e. the last few degrees of flexion) cannot be carried out (loss Illus.) physiotherapy should be considered.

40. Need for rehabilitation (b): 2. Assess the patient's grip strength by first asking her to squeeze two of your fingers as tightly as possible while you try to withdraw them. Compare one hand with the other. Repeat with a single finger. Marked weakness is an indication for physiotherapy.

41. Need for rehabilitation (c): 3. Assess wrist movements. Initially, material restriction of *palmar flexion* is normal and by itself is of little importance. If, however, the total range of *pronation and supination* is less than half normal, physiotherapy is advisable. 4. Where there is only slight restriction of movements and power, rehabilitation may still be indicated through the special requirements of the patient's work.

42. Alternative fixation methods (a): A Pennig Dynamic Wrist Fixator may be used where the fracture cannot be satisfactorily reduced or held by closed methods. Where the distal radial fragment is intact or occasionally with an undisplaced intra-articular fracture (AO = A2.2, A3.2, C1.2) pins are inserted in the distal fragment and the radial shaft. After assembly of the fixator, the fracture is reduced and the clamp screws locked. The wrist can be mobilised immediately.

43. Alternative fixation methods (b): Where there is severe comminution (Illus.), or splitting of the radial fragment into two or more displaced fragments an external fixator may also be used to bridge the fracture and the wrist joint. The distal pins are usually placed in the shaft of the second metacarpal. This allows control of length while avoiding the necessity of having to put the wrist up in marked flexion to maintain the reduction.

44. Alternative fixation methods (c): Where during a manipulative procedure instability is found to be marked, and it is considered that it will be very difficult to maintain any reduction with a cast alone, then the position may be stabilised with Kirschner wires. The most secure and reliable configuration[1] is thought to be that of Kapandji (modified by Fritz et al) where a third K-wire is used. (Where this should be positioned is indicated by the dotted line on the radiograph above.) An additional plaster cast will be required until union of the fracture is well advanced. The wires may be removed after 3-4 weeks. In similar circumstances, plating of the fracture may also be considered. Anterior plates are most commonly used. A word of caution: the use of K-wires has been shown in the long term to offer no more than a marginal improvement on the radiographic appearances and overall function.[2]

45. Splitting of the radial fragment (a): There may be a small vertical crack through the radial fragment, showing in the AP view (1). In others the fracture may run horizontally, and the scaphoid or lunate may separate the fragments (2). In the young adult, especially where the main fragments are separated and there is no gross fragmentation, internal fixation is indicated. (Barton's fracture (see Frame 75) is similar, but with an intact posterior radial buttress.)

46. Splitting of the radial fragment (b): In a number of cases the fracture may be reduced under intensifier control (or under vision using an arthroscope). Kirschner wires may be used to lever the fragments into position prior to the insertion of the Kirschner fixation wires which are shown in this radiograph. Additional support with a cast will be needed. Some permanent joint stiffness is the rule after injuries of this pattern, and prolonged physiotherapy will usually be required.

47. Splitting of the radial fragment (c): Where comminution is not a problem, the distal fragments may be approximated with a cross screw (indicated by an arrow in the illustration). The distal radius may then be aligned with the shaft and held with a plate and screws. In this case a dorsal plate has been employed.

48. Splitting of the radial fragment (d): More commonly a pre-contoured volar plate may be used. This is first attached to the distal fragment with locking screws, resulting in the stem of the plate standing proud of the radial shaft. Levering it back into contact with the anterior surface of the radial shaft then leads to correction of the anterior angulation deformity. This technique may also be used with Colles pattern fractures uncomplicated by splitting of the distal fragment.

49. Splitting of the radial fragment (e): In some cases the degree of comminution or softness of the bone texture may render screw fixation in the distal fragments ineffective. In the case illustrated, although there are two reasonably substantial distal fragments, the horizontal line of the fracture is close to the joint leaving little bone for screw fixation. There is an additional vertical split in the radius.

50. Splitting of the radial fragment (f): In these circumstances the fracture was brought to length using a Pennig fixator, with pins in the radius and index metacarpal. The fragment which includes the styloid process was secured using two Kirschner wires, while the smaller medial fragment was held with an additional K-wire.

51. Complications (a): Persistent deformity or mal-union (i): Radial drift of the distal fragment results in prominence of the distal radius (1). Radial tilting and bony absorption at the fracture site lead to relative prominence of the distal ulna (2) and tilting of the plane of the wrist as seen in the AP radiographs (3). These deformities may be symptom free, and surgery on purely cosmetic grounds is seldom indicated.

52. Mal-union (ii): In some cases there is quite marked pain in the region of the distal radio-ulnar joint, owing to its severe disorganisation. There is generally quite *marked local tenderness* and supination in particular is reduced. Physiotherapy in the form of grip strengthening and pronation/supination exercises is indicated. If symptoms remain severe, excision of the distal end of the ulna may be considered.

53. Mal-union (iii): Uncomplicated persistence of dinner-fork deformity (i.e. persistent deformity in the lateral but not in the AP radiographs) is accompanied by some loss of palmar flexion, but significant functional disturbance is unusual. This type of residual deformity is generally accepted.

54. Complications (b): *Delayed rupture of extensor pollicis longus* may follow Colles fracture, and be due to attrition of the tendon by roughness at the fracture site, or by sloughing from interference with its blood supply. Disability is often slight, and spontaneous recovery may occur. There is no urgency regarding treatment, and in the elderly this complaint may be accepted or treated expectantly. In the young, an extensor indicis proprius tendon transfer is advocated.

55. Complications (c): Sudeck's atrophy/complex regional pain syndrome: This is often detected about the time the patient comes out of plaster. The fingers are swollen and finger flexion is restricted. The hand and wrist are warm, tender and painful. Radiographs show diffuse osteoporosis (Illus.). *Treatment.* (1) The mainstay of treatment is intensive and prolonged physiotherapy and occupational therapy, but (2) if pain is very severe a further 2-3 weeks rest of the *wrist* in plaster may give sufficient relief to allow commencement of effective finger movements. (3) If the MP joints are stiff in extension and making no headway, manipulation under general anaesthesia followed by fixation in plaster (MP joints flexed, IP joints extended) for 3 weeks only may be effective in initiating recovery. (4) In severe cases, a sympathetic block may be attempted by infiltration of the stellate ganglion. (See Ch. 5 for a fuller discussion.)

56. Complications (d): Carpal tunnel (median nerve compression) syndrome: Paraesthesiae in the median distribution is the main presenting symptom, but look for sensory and motor involvement. *If detected before reduction:* (i) Complete lesion: reduce, plaster and re-assess. If no improvement, explore, and divide not only the roof of the carpal tunnel but the antebrachial fascia. (ii) Partial lesion: reduce and apply a cast; if motor symptoms remain, or if symptoms persist for a week, decompress.

57. Median nerve compression syndrome *ctd:* *If detected after reduction:* Release the splints, put the wrist in the neutral position, and use Kirschner wires or an external fixator to hold the reduction; if symptoms persist, explore. *If detected after union:* Exploration is generally advised, as symptoms otherwise tend to persist. Note that the diagnosis at the late stage may be suggested by the response to tapping over the nerve (Illus.), or by nerve stretching, tourniquet, or nerve conduction tests.

58. Complications (e): Persisting stiffness: Restriction of movements, even after prolonged physiotherapy, is not uncommon, but is seldom severe enough to impair limb function to a material extent. This is due to compensatory (trick) movements developed by the elbow, shoulder and trunk (e.g. in case of loss of supination).

59. Complications (f): Associated scaphoid fracture: This may be treated by manipulation of the Colles fracture and application of a scaphoid plaster. After the Colles fracture has united, further immobilisation may be required for the scaphoid. Alternatively, the scaphoid fracture may be fixed with an AO lag cancellous screw (Illus.) (or a Herbert screw), the Colles fracture manipulated, and fixation discontinued as soon as the latter has united.

60. Related fractures (a): A number of fractures involving the distal end of the radius, produced by falls on the outstretched hand, have certain similarities to the classical Colles fracture. The commonest of these is the *undisplaced greenstick fracture of the radius.* In its most minor form it may be overlooked; the only sign may be slight local buckling. These are sometimes referred to as torus or buckle fractures.

61. Undisplaced greenstick fracture of the radius *ctd:* The level of the fracture is variable, and it may be situated fairly proximally. This type of fracture may be treated by the application of a plaster slab, completed after 1-2 days, and retained for about 3 weeks. This fracture may also be treated successfully with an off-the-shelf brace. The Futura wrist splint, which is held in position with Velcro fasteners, is perhaps the most popular of these devices.

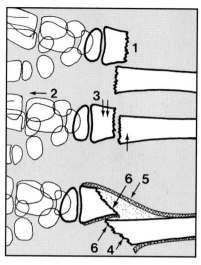

62. Related fracture (b): Angled greenstick fracture of the radius: In this type of injury there is both clinical and radiological deformity. Manipulation is required as for a Colles fracture, and the aftercare is similar; the period of plaster fixation may be reduced to 3 or 4 weeks, depending on the age of the child.

63. Related fractures (c): Overlapping radial fracture: In children the radius often fractures close to the wrist, with off-ending (i.e. complete loss of bony contact). On the ulnar side there may be: 1. detachment of the triangular fibrocartilage; 2. separation of the ulnar epiphysis; 3. fracture and angulation of the distal ulna; 4. fracture and displacement of the distal ulna (Illus.), in effect a fracture of both bones of the forearm; 5. dislocation of the ulna (Galeazzi fracture-dislocation).

64. Overlapping radial fracture *ctd:* If the fracture line is transverse (1), reduction is straightforward by traction (2) and local pressure (3). When, however, there is a fracture running obliquely forward from front to back (4), reduction by traction is often impossible owing to the integrity of the periosteum on the dorsal surface (5) and the overlapping bony spikes (6).

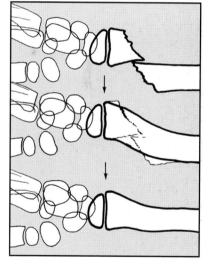

65. Overlapping radial fracture *ctd:* Two closed techniques may be tried. For the first, two assistants are essential to apply *maximal* traction to the limb (1). While this is being strongly maintained, the surgeon should press forcibly with the heel of one hand on the distal fragment (2) and use the other to apply counter-pressure (3). Reduction is achieved by shearing off one of the bone spikes (4).

66. Overlapping radial fracture *ctd:* Alternatively, by *increasing* the deformity (1) and applying pressure directly over the distal radial fragment (2), whilst maintaining traction (3), reduction may be achieved. After the fragments have interlocked the angulation is corrected. Thereafter plaster fixation is carried out as in other fractures in this region.

67. Overlapping radial fracture *ctd:* If shortening is marked, and closed methods fail, open reduction may be considered. (Performed through a small dorsal incision under a tourniquet; internal fixation is not required, although a Kirschner wire may be used to hold the fracture temporarily - being withdrawn as soon as the plaster has been applied.) Nevertheless, if persisting overlap is reluctantly accepted, a good result from remodelling is the usual outcome (Illus.) *provided* any angulation is corrected.

68. Related fractures (d): Slipped radial epiphysis: This injury is common in adolescence, and the displaced distal radial epiphysis is usually associated with a small fracture of the metaphysis (Salter-Harris Type 2 injury). Unless displacement is minimal, manipulation followed by plaster fixation (as for a Colles fracture) is indicated. Growth disturbance is rare, but reduction should be carried out promptly (it is often difficult to reduce after 2 days).

69. Related fractures (e): Fracture of the radial styloid: This fracture may be caused by an engine starting-handle kickback (the so-called 'chauffeur's fracture') or by a fall on the outstretched hand. Displacement is usually slight, and manipulation is unlikely to be of value. Every case should be checked for scapho-lunate dissociation. A Colles plaster is usually adequate, although some prefer fixation with a lag screw or Kirschner wires. Physiotherapy is usually required, and Sudeck's atrophy a common complication.

70. Related fractures (f): Smith's fracture (i): This injury frequently results from a fall on the back of the hand, although a clear history is not always obtainable. The distal radial fragment is tilted anteriorly (posterior angulation) and may be displaced anteriorly. The fracture is usually impacted. Greenstick fractures of this pattern are common.

71. Smith's fracture (ii): This fracture is frequently referred to as a reversed Colles fracture, because the deformities when viewed from the side are in the opposite direction to those seen in a Colles fracture. (Note, however, that the two fractures may be identical in AP radiographs.) Comminuted Smith's fractures may involve the articular surface of the radius (Illus.). *Adult fractures are best treated by the application of a volar plate.*

72. Smith's fracture (iii): As an alternative to surgery (e.g. in children or where the patient, because of other injuries or poor health, is unfit for prolonged anaesthesia) these fractures may be treated conservatively. Traction is first applied to the arm (1) in supination (2) until disimpaction is achieved. (This may be confirmed as in a Colles fracture.) Pressure may be applied with the heels of the hands to force the distal fragment dorsally (3).

73. Smith's fracture (iv): The reduction is difficult to hold, and a long arm plaster is required (1). This may be more conveniently applied in two stages, and a complete plaster is better than a simple slab. The arm is held in full supination and dorsiflexion (2). This is easily maintained with the elbow extended (3). The arm is measured for an anterior forearm slab (4) and wool roll applied to the arm.

74. Smith's fracture (v): The anterior slab is trimmed (5) and positioned (6) before completion of the forearm part of the cast (7) which may be moulded while setting. The cast is then extended above the elbow. *Aftercare:* Split if necessary; radiographs at weekly intervals for the first 3 weeks (treat any slipping by remanipulation or moulding); change slack plasters with care. Six weeks' fixation is usually required, with physiotherapy after removal of the cast.

75. Related fractures (g): Barton's fracture: This is a form of Smith's fracture in which the anterior portion only of the radius is involved. Closed reduction may be attempted along the lines indicated for Smith's fracture, but this often fails with the carpus wedging the fragments apart.

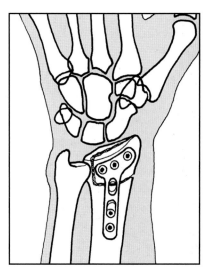

76. Barton's fracture *ctd:* In the young patient these potentially unstable and disabling fractures are therefore best treated by open reduction and internal fixation. The most satisfactory procedure is to expose the fracture anteriorly and reduce it under vision; thereafter it is best held with a volar plate (e.g. with an LCP radius plate, a buttress plate, or an AO right angled or oblique T-plate (Illus.)).

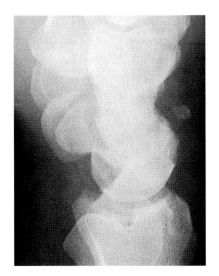

77. Related fractures (h): Forcible palmar flexion may result in a *minor avulsion fracture of the carpus* at a ligament insertion (Illus.). If the wrist is forcibly palmar flexed or dorsiflexed, the carpus impinging on the distal end of the radius may produce a *marginal chip fracture of the radius.* Symptomatic treatment only is required for any of these injuries (e.g. 2-3 weeks in a plaster back slab).

78. Fractures of the scaphoid: Mechanisms of injury: Scaphoid fractures often result from 'kickback' when using starting handles on internal combustion generators, pumps, compressors and inboard marine engines. (The motorist's avoidance of this fracture is his only dividend from the unfortunate abolition of car starting handles.) Otherwise the fracture may be acquired by falls on the outstretched hand.

79. Fractures of the scaphoid: Diagnosis (a): Fracture of the scaphoid may be suspected when there is complaint of pain on the lateral aspect of the wrist following any injury (or frequently repeated stress). In those cases which follow starting handle accidents there may be marked and rapid swelling of the hand and wrist.

80. Diagnosis (b): Tenderness in the anatomical snuff box (1) is suggestive of this injury, but by no means diagnostic. Many wrist sprains without fracture give rise to tenderness in this site. Beware too of tenderness which may be the result of a Bennett's fracture of the thumb metacarpal (2) or of a fracture of the radial styloid (3).

81. Diagnosis (c): In a true scaphoid fracture, tenderness will also be elicited on the application of pressure over the *dorsal aspect of the scaphoid*, and also on pressure over the palmar aspect. Tenderness in these additional sites very seldom occurs in other injuries in this area, no matter how severe.

82. Diagnosis (d): Radiographs (i): Radiography is required in all suspect cases. Note the following important points:
(1) Request cards should be clearly marked 'scaphoid' and not 'wrist'. This is necessary to ensure that the films are properly centred, and that at least three projections of the scaphoid are obtained to improve the chances of the fracture being visualised in the initial radiographic series.
(2) The fracture is often hairline, and as a consequence hard to detect.
(3) Because of this accepted difficulty - i.e. that a hairline fracture may not show up on the initial films - it is common practice in all suspected but unconfirmed cases that radiographs should be repeated at 10-14 days. Although there is some controversy about this, the common view is that local decalcification after such an interval may reveal a previously hidden fracture.
(4) Alternatively, and if the facilities are available, high resolution multi-slice CT scans and/or 3-D reconstruction may resolve the problem.
(5) In some cases a bone scan may be helpful. Note that there is a 20% rate of false positive reporting of scaphoid radiographs, and *clinical confirmation of the diagnosis is mandatory*.

83. Radiographs (ii): This radiograph is typical of a fracture through the waist of the scaphoid. In this example the fracture line is easily seen in both the AP projection and one oblique - but this by no means is always the case.

84. Anatomical features (a): The scaphoid (shaded) plays a key role in wrist and carpal function, taking part in the radiocarpal joint (1) and in the joint between the proximal and distal rows of the carpus (2). It articulates with the radius (R), trapezium (Tm), trapezoid (Td), capitate (C) and lunate (L). The commonest site for fracture is the waist (50%); 38% of fractures occur in the proximal half and 12% in the distal half. (U = ulna, H = hamate, P = pisiform, Tl = triquetral.)

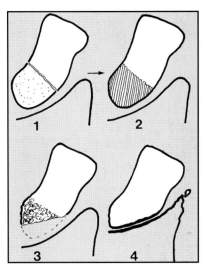

85. Anatomical features (b): A number of abnormalities in ossification may be confused with fractures. The *os centrale* may be small (1), large (2) or double (3). The *os radiale externum* (4) lies in the region of the tubercle and in some cases may represent an old, ununited fracture; certainly the so-called 'bipartite scaphoid' (5) is now generally regarded as being due to this. (Rounded edges differentiate these from fresh fractures.)

86. Anatomical features (c): The blood supply of the scaphoid is through small vessels which enter the ligamentous ridge (1) lying between the two main articular surfaces (2). When these vessels are well scattered (a), ischaemia following fracture is uncommon. If all the vessels enter the distal part of the ridge (b), fractures of the waist (W) and proximal poles (P) may be followed by avascular necrosis.

87. Anatomical features (d): Avascular necrosis is of immediate onset, but 1-2 months may elapse before increased bone density betrays its presence on the radiographs (2). There is usually slow but progressive bony collapse (3) and radiocarpal osteoarthritis (4). This leads to worsening pain and stiffness in the wrist. Avascular necrosis occurs in about 30% of fractures of the proximal pole of the scaphoid.

88. Anatomical features (e): Because of its role in two major joints (1), movement of the fragments is difficult to control, and non-union may occur in waist fractures. Cystic changes at the fracture site (2) are followed by marginal sclerosis (3). The edges may round off and form a symptomless pseudarthrosis (4) or osteoarthritis may supervene (5). Note that non-union can occur without avascular necrosis, and that most fractures with avascular necrosis are united.

89. Prognostic features: The prognosis is good in *stable* injuries: these include (Herbert Classification) fractures of the tubercle (A1), and hairline fractures of the waist (A2). The prognosis is poorer in *unstable* injuries which include oblique fractures of the distal third (B1), displaced fractures of the waist (B2), proximal pole fractures (B3), fractures associated with carpal dislocations (B4) (Illus.: trans-scapho perilunar dislocation of the carpus - see Frame 109) and comminuted fractures (B5).

90. Treatment of suspected fracture: When there is local tenderness and normal radiographs, apply a scaphoid plaster and sling. Remove the plaster and re-X-ray at 2 weeks (see also Frame 82). Absorption of bone at the site of any hairline fracture will then usually reveal it. If a fracture is confirmed, apply a fresh cast and treat as for a frank fracture. If the radiographs are negative, the patient is presumed to have suffered a sprain, and is treated accordingly: but if symptoms persist re-examine and X-ray after another 2 weeks.

91. Fractures of the tuberosity of the scaphoid: Avascular necrosis never occurs in fractures of this type, and non-union here does not give rise to significant symptoms. Symptomatic treatment only is needed (e.g. a crepe bandage or plaster, depending on pain). Some extend this to include all distal pole fractures, but generally plaster fixation is the mainstay of treatment of these fractures.

92. Treatment of undisplaced fractures of the waist of the scaphoid (a): The long established practice has been to treat undisplaced fractures of the waist of the scaphoid by cast fixation until the fracture has united or until there is evidence of non-union. (Union is reported as occurring within 6-8 weeks in 85-95% of patients treated conservatively.)

Many, however, advocate internal fixation of all fractures of this pattern. After an initial period of protection this certainly avoids 4 or more weeks in a cast, but it has been shown that there is a 15% complication rate and no other significant advantage (apart from some advance in starting treatment of non-union should this ensue). In order to avoid over treatment of a large proportion of fractures and subjugating patients to avoidable surgical risks Dias[3] advocates plaster fixation for 6-8 weeks followed by plain films, and if there is doubt, CT scans. Only if a gap is then demonstrated should internal fixation, with or without bone grafting, be carried out. This should ensure union in 95% of cases. Unless there are commanding reasons for internal fixation in a particular case this would seem to be a reasoned approach and in consequence the following section deals with the application of a scaphoid plaster.

93. Treatment of undisplaced fractures of the waist of the scaphoid (b): The classical scaphoid plaster (i): The position of the hand is of some importance and should be made quite clear to the patient prior to the application of the plaster. In the classical scaphoid plaster (a position nevertheless challenged by some) the wrist should be fully pronated (1), radially deviated (2), and moderately dorsiflexed (3). In addition, the thumb should be in mid abduction (4).

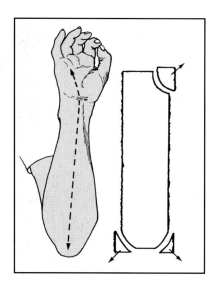

94. The scaphoid plaster (ii): An anterior plaster slab, although by no means essential, is frequently used. This may be made from 6-8 layers of 10 cm (4″) plaster bandage, or taken from a slab dispenser. The proximal corners should be trimmed and a cut-out made to accommodate the swell of the thenar muscles.

95. The scaphoid plaster (iii): Stockingette is applied from just above the elbow (1) to the proximal phalanges (2), allowing for subsequent turn-down. A smaller gauge (or wool roll) may be used for the thumb (3). A turn of wool is used to protect the bony prominences of the wrist (4). If there is a lot of early swelling suggesting more to come, more generous wool padding is applied round the wrist and hand.

96. The scaphoid plaster (iv): The plaster slab may then be wetted and applied to the forearm, taking care not to extend it beyond the proximal palmar crease (5). Encircling plaster bandages are then applied, using 15 cm (6″) bandages for the forearm, 10 cm (4″) for the wrist and 7.5 cm (3″) for the thumb (6). The edges of the stockingette are turned down before completion (7).

97. The scaphoid plaster (v): Common faults: Plaster including MP joints of fingers, restricting flexion (1). Terminal phalanx of thumb included, preventing interphalangeal joint flexion (2). Plaster too short (3). Plaster restricting flexion of the elbow (4). (Note that to give the best support to a scaphoid fracture there is some questioning of the position of the wrist and the need to include the thumb. Some use a Colles plaster in neutral or slight flexion, without radial deviation.)

98. Scaphoid fracture: Aftercare (a): A sling should be worn for the first few days until swelling subsides. Analgesics are usually required initially. The patient is reviewed at 2 weeks (assuming the initial plaster check has been satisfactory). If on this visit the plaster is unduly slack, it should be changed. Any softening in the palm should be reinforced.

99. Aftercare (b): At 6 weeks the plaster should be removed and the scaphoid assessed clinically and with radiographs. There are several possibilities: (i) if there is no tenderness over the dorsal surface and in the snuff-box, and the fracture appears united on the radiographs, the wrist should be left free and reviewed in 2 weeks (usually for discharge, or further radiographs if pain recurs).

100. Aftercare (c): (ii) The fracture line may still show clearly on the radiographs. (iii) The radiographs may suggest union, but there is marked local tenderness. (iv) There is some uncertainty on either score. These possibilities are all suggestive of delayed union, and a further 6 weeks of plaster fixation is desirable. If, however, there is a clear *gap*, see Frame 102.

101. Aftercare (d): At 12 weeks, there may be: (i) evidence of *avascular necrosis* (Illustrated: note the increase in the density of the proximal half of the scaphoid in this radiograph), (ii) clear evidence, clinically and radiologically of *union*. In these circumstances, there is no need and no advantage in continuing with plaster fixation.

102. Aftercare (e): Note at 12 weeks (or preferably at 6 weeks) if there is evidence of a gap between the scaphoid fragments. If there is any doubt, an MRI scan (Illus.) may help clarify this. The appearance of a gap is a significant finding, as if it is not acted upon there is a significant increase in the chances of non-union.

103. Aftercare (f): .A gap is an indication for internal fixation, and the larger it is or the later it is detected, the greater the need for a supplementary bone graft. To hold the fracture, small cancellous bone screws may be used, but the most popular devices incorporate dual pitch screw threads, the effect of which is to draw the fragments together as the screws become fully engaged. Illustrated is an Acutrak dual pitch screw; this is cannulated so that it may be inserted percutaneously.

104. Displaced fracture of the scaphoid (i): If there is marked displacement (Illus.), be sure to exclude a concurrent carpal dislocation. Where displacement or angulation exceed 1 mm or 15° respectively, internal fixation is indicated; indeed, as the results of internal fixation are so very good, many advocate this for every displaced scaphoid fracture.

105. Displaced fracture of the scaphoid (ii): The illustration shows a fracture of the scaphoid held with a dual pitch Herbert screw. The case was one of a displaced fracture through the waist of the scaphoid and part of a trans-scapho perilunar dislocation of the wrist (see 3, Frame 109); the Kirschner wires have been inserted to stabilise the reduction of the carpal dislocation.

(c) If an early impingement osteoarthritis threatens, satisfactory results may be obtained from excision of the radial styloid even although the midcarpal joint is unaffected by this (Illus.).
(d) Symptomless non-union of the scaphoid, sometimes discovered by accident, should have the risks of secondary osteoarthritis assessed; if the appearances indicate that these are insignificant, then no treatment is indicated.

108. Complications (d): Advanced osteoarthritis: This generally occurs as a sequel to avascular necrosis or non-union. The following treatments may be considered:
1. Wrist joint (radiocarpal) fusion: Pronation and supination movements are retained, but all other wrist movements are lost. This is the most reliable procedure and is the only one which should be pursued in the patient who undertakes heavy manual labour.
2. Where the retention of some wrist movement is essential, excision of the proximal row of the carpus may be considered. The results are a little unpredictable in terms of the final range of movements, strength, and freedom from pain.
3. Where surgery is thought inadvisable, good results in terms of relief from pain, with reasonable function may be obtained by the use of a block-leather support, or similar orthotic device.

106. Complications (a): Sudeck's atrophy/ complex regional pain syndrome: Treat as described in Frame 55.
(b) Avascular necrosis: In the early stages an anterior bone block graft (e.g. Matti-Russe operation) may be considered. In the late stages where is bony collapse (Illus.) only salvage procedures (such as those detailed in Frame 108) are likely to be of benefit.

107. Complications (c): Non-union: (a) It is reported that late diagnosed non-union, seen 3-6 months after injury, may still be effectively treated by plaster fixation and pulsed magnetic fields, *provided* that there is no displacement, carpal collapse, or osteoarthritic change.
(b) If there is displacement, or if seen later than 6 months, and symptoms are present, internal fixation and bone grafting are advised.

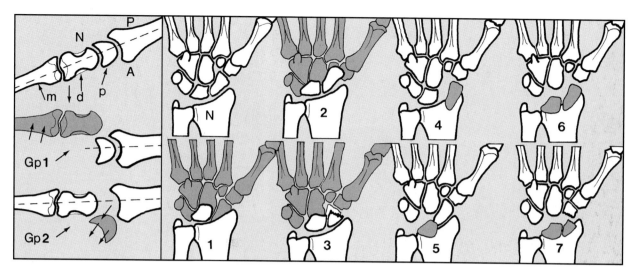

109. Dislocations of the carpus: These may result from a fall on the outstretched hand, and are comparatively uncommon. There are two main groups. In the first, the metacarpals (m), the distal row of the carpus (d) and part of the proximal row (p) dislocate backwards. In classifying injuries within this group, the prefix 'peri' is used to describe undisplaced structures in the proximal row. Occasionally one of the carpal bones fractures, part remaining in alignment and part displacing with the distal row of the carpus. Note in the illustrations that structures drawn in faint lines and shaded in dark grey are *displaced* (N = normal appearance from the side or *volar* aspect): (1) perilunar dislocation of the carpus; (2) periscapholunar dislocation of the carpus; (3) trans-scapho perilunar dislocation of the carpus. (Not illustrated are the rare transcapitate, transtriquetral perilunar dislocations and others.) In the second main group of injuries, the distal row re-aligns with the radius and part of the proximal row is extruded: hence: (4) dislocation of the scaphoid; (5) dislocation of the lunate; (6) dislocation of the lunate and scaphoid; (7) dislocation of the lunate and part of the scaphoid. (Note the correspondence between 1 and 5, 2 and 6, 3 and 7.)

110. Dislocation of the lunate: This is the commonest of all the carpal dislocations, and generally results from a fall on the outstretched hand. It is frequently overlooked, and this is nearly always due to failure in interpretation of the radiographs. Note in the normal radiographs of the carpus (Illus.) that the pisiform bone stands out to a varying degree from the rest of the volar surface.

111. Dislocation of the lunate: The *shape* of the dislocated lunate is quite different from the ovoid/quadrilateral mass of the pisiform. The *concave surface* in which the capitate usually sits is *rotated* anteriorly, and the crescent moon shape of the bone (and hence its name) is rendered obvious. The articular surfaces of the scaphoid and triquetral remain aligned with the radius while the lunate is *displaced* anteriorly. In the AP projection, the lunate is sector-shaped (resembling a cheese segment). *Diagnosis:* This is established on the basis of a history of injury, local tenderness and the radiographs. Evidence of median nerve involvement is very suggestive; this may result from direct pressure of the displaced bone on the nerve.

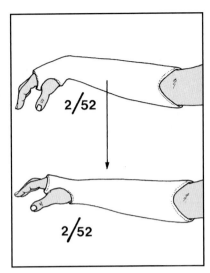

112. Treatment (a): Reduction can generally be achieved by closed methods under general anaesthesia. (1) Apply traction to the supinated wrist. (2) Extend the wrist, maintaining traction. (3) Apply pressure with the thumb over the lunate. (4) Flex the wrist as soon as you feel the lunate slip into position.

113. Treatment (b): Alternatively, if an assistant is available, he should apply traction in supination and extension as before (1) while you use both thumbs to push the lunate posteriorly and distally (2). When it is felt to reduce, the wrist is once again flexed. The reduction should be checked with radiographs before the anaesthetic is discontinued. (Failure is an indication for open reduction.)

114. Treatment (c): (i) The wrist is encased in plaster in a position of moderate flexion for 1-2 weeks. (ii) The plaster is then changed for one with the wrist in the neutral position for a further 2 weeks. (iii) Weekly radiographs should be taken to detect any late subluxation (an indication for K-wire fixation). (iv) Physiotherapy may be required, depending on the degree of residual stiffness. Swelling may be a problem initially, and require generous padding, elevation, and a sling.

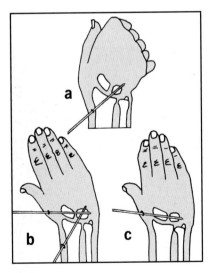

115. Treatment (d): Many prefer K-wire fixation in all cases. To do this the wrist is put in flexion and full ulnar deviation, and the lunate fixed to the radius with a K-wire (a). The wrist is then positioned in dorsiflexion and radial deviation and a second wire passed through the scaphoid into the lunate (b). The wrist is then placed in a more neutral position and the first wire removed. A light cast is worn for 5-6 weeks. The wire is retained for 4 weeks.

116. Complications (a): Late diagnosis: If there is delay in making the diagnosis, manipulative reduction becomes increasingly difficult, and after a week may not be possible. Open reduction is then necessary, and carries with it the greatly increased risk of avascular necrosis. Surgery should be performed through an anterior incision, and every effort made to reduce the bone without disturbing any of its ligamentous attachments (evidence suggests the major blood supply enters anteriorly) or further damaging the median nerve.

(b) Median nerve palsy: Prompt reduction of the dislocation is usually followed by early complete recovery. After late reduction recovery may be incomplete, but seldom requires separate treatment.

(c) Sudeck's atrophy/complex regional pain syndrome: This is a common complication and is treated along previously described lines.

(d) Avascular necrosis: (Illus.). This leads to collapse of the lunate and secondary osteoarthritis which advances with great rapidity. *All cases of dislocated lunate should have monthly radiographs for 6 months* to allow early detection of this complication. If detected early, excision may prevent progressive osteoarthritis. In many cases, and certainly at the later stages, arthrodesis of the wrist is preferable.

Note that repeated trauma to the wrist without frank dislocation of the lunate may lead to similar radiographic appearances (Kienbock's disease); this condition is found in manual workers such as carpenters, cobblers and jack hammer (pneumatic drill) operators.

117. Dislocation and subluxation of the scaphoid (see also Carpal Instability and Scapholunate Dissociation) (a): These uncommon injuries are diagnosed radiologically and, if suspected, AP projections in both radial and ulnar deviation may be helpful. The most striking feature is the widening of the space between the scaphoid and lunate.

Treatment: 1. If the displacement is anterior and complete as shown, manipulate as for dislocation of the lunate. 2. In many cases, dislocation is incomplete, with the proximal pole being tilted posteriorly and the distal pole anteriorly. Such injuries have often a toggle-like instability within the dorsiflexion/palmar flexion range (and the stable position within this phase must be found by trial and error during reduction). (See also Frame 124.)

118. (b) *ctd:* Reduction may be achieved by pressure over the proximal pole. If possible, an image intensifier should be used to check the reduction and stability. If a stable position is found, the wrist should be put up in plaster in that position, with some radial deviation; the plaster should be retained for 6 weeks, with frequent radiographs to check the position. If instability is not easily controlled, then the scaphoid should certainly be fixed with Kirschner wires, a procedure many advocate for all cases. Many prefer primary internal fixation of the scaphoid in all injuries of this pattern.

119. Dislocation of the lunate and half the scaphoid: This combination of injuries may be treated by manipulative reduction as described for dislocation of the lunate. Thereafter it is probably best to internally fix the scaphoid fracture, e.g. with a Herbert screw. These injuries have a much poorer prognosis than uncomplicated dislocations of the lunate.

120. Trans-scapho perilunar dislocation of the carpus: This injury corresponds to dislocation of the lunate and half the scaphoid just described. It is the commonest of the first group of carpal dislocations. In some cases there may be associated fractures of the styloid process of the radius and the ulna. Treatment: reduction by traction is usually easy. Thereafter the management is that of fracture of the scaphoid. If, however, the scaphoid reduction is poor or if the wrist is very unstable, internal fixation of the scaphoid and stabilisation of the carpus (e.g. by Kirschner wires) must be considered.

121. Other carpal injuries (a): Perilunar dislocation of the carpus: This corresponds to isolated dislocation of the lunate.
Treatment: 1. Reduce by traction.
2. Apply a plaster cast with the wrist in flexion and retain for 1-2 weeks before
3. changing the plaster to one with the wrist in the neutral position. This should be retained for a further 2 weeks.
4. Thereafter physiotherapy may be required to mobilise the wrist.

122. Other carpal injuries *ctd:* (b) Dislocation of both the lunate and scaphoid: This should be treated as for dislocation of the lunate.
(c) Periscapholunar dislocation of the carpus: This should be treated in the same way as perilunar dislocation of the carpus.
(d) Dislocation of the trapezium, trapezoid or hamate: These are rare. Closed reduction should always be attempted, but open reduction is frequently required. In the face of instability, transfixion by Kirschner wires may be helpful.
(e) Fractures through the bodies of any of the carpal bones other than the scaphoid: These are rare, and should be treated symptomatically by 6 weeks' fixation in a Colles or scaphoid plaster (depending on the injury). Fractures of the hamate (see also below) and pisiform may be complicated by ulnar nerve palsy, which should generally be treated expectantly.
(f) Small chip fractures of the carpus: These are common and usually result from hyperflexion or hyperextension injuries of the wrist. Direct violence is sometimes responsible. The bone of origin is often in doubt. Rest of the wrist in plaster for 3 weeks is all that is required, and full recovery of function is the rule.

123. Other carpal injuries *ctd:* (g) Fracture of the hook of the hamate: This injury is seen most often as a result of a heavy golf or tennis swing, but may follow a fall, or a direct blow in the palm. There is local pain and tenderness. The fracture is best shown by a CT scan of both wrists in the praying position (1), or by carpal tunnel films (2). The best treatment is to excise the hamate fragment. (h = hamate; c = capitate; t = trapezium; S = scaphoid; P = pisiform; Q = triquetral; L = lunate)

124. Carpal instabilities: A carpal instability is a condition in which there is a loss of normal carpal alignment that develops at an early or late stage after an injury.
In *static carpal instabilities* there is an abnormal carpal alignment which can be seen by careful study of standard AP and lateral radiographs of the wrist. In *dorsiflexion instability* the lunate is rotated into dorsiflexion; in *palmar flexion instability* the lunate is rotated into palmar flexion; in *ulnar translocation* the whole carpus is displaced in an ulnar direction; and in *dorsal subluxation* the carpus in displaced in a dorsal direction.
In *dynamic carpal instabilities* routine radiographs are normal. The patient is usually able to toggle his carpal alignment from normal to abnormal and back, or manipulation of the scaphoid by the examiner may reproduce the sensation of instability of which the patient usually complains. To establish the diagnosis, place lead markers on the skin over points of local tenderness, and take radiographs in both stable and unstable positions.

In the case of scapholunate instability, AP views of the supinated wrist in both radial and ulnar deviation are usually diagnostic. Examination of the wrist in motion using an image intensifier may also be helpful. Other investigations: 1. A radio-isotope bone scan may be carried out. If this is negative, either the diagnosis is incorrect, or local inflammatory changes are of such a minor degree that no more than conservative management should be considered.
2. Ultrasound may be used. 3. MRI scans and arthrography may be helpful in detecting the presence and location of (intercarpal) ligament tears. The commonest instability is between the *scaphoid and lunate* (scapholunate dissociation) (Illus.). If untreated this may be followed by osteoarthritis.

Treatment: 1. In the acute case: manipulative reduction using the image intensifier, followed by the insertion of K-wires. The technique is similar to that used for dislocation of the lunate: in the example shown two K-wires have been used for better carpal fixation. *Alternatively* an open repair of the torn ligaments may be undertaken. 2. In chronic cases, reattachment of the avulsed scapholunate ligament may be carried out, but where there are arthritic changes and subluxation a salvage procedure may have to be considered.

125. Injuries to the metacarpals and phalanges - general principles: In assessing how best to treat a specific injury, begin by making sure there is no significant soft-tissue involvement such as nerve or tendon injury, or substantial skin loss (see later for further details). Next, from the radiographs, assess whether the bony alignment can be judged as being acceptable. (Illus.: acceptable undisplaced fractures of the shafts of the middle and ring metacarpals.)

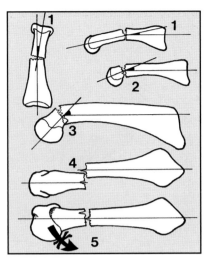

126. Assessing position *ctd:* Generally speaking, the position of a metacarpal or phalangeal fracture can be considered acceptable (i) if angulation does not exceed 10° in either the lateral or AP projections (1): but in the lateral, 20° may be accepted in the metaphysis (2) and 45° in the neck of the fifth metacarpal (3); (ii) if there is at least 50% bony contact (4); (iii) if there is no rotational deformity (5).

127. Assessing position *ctd:* Rotational deformity may not always be obvious on the radiographs, or clinically when a finger is in the extended position. Note, however, that when the fingers are individually flexed that they all touch the palm close to the scaphoid. Check that this is the case. (The same precaution should be taken when the quality of a reduction is being assessed or when splintage is being applied.)

128. Assessing stability: Now go on and make an assessment of the *stability* of the fracture. Undisplaced transverse and longitudinal fractures are generally *stable*, but the following are usually *unstable:* (1) rotated spiral and some oblique fractures; (2) multifragmentary fractures; (3) severely displaced fractures; (4) multiple fractures; (5) fractures through the neck of a proximal phalanx; (6) displaced articular fractures.

129. Assessing stability *ctd:* If there is some remaining doubt, assess the *functional stability* of the fracture. This is done by asking the patient to flex the injured finger (without assistance) and assessing the range of movements in the joints on either side of the fracture. If the fracture is functionally stable the range obtained should reach 30% of the normal range, (i.e. MP = 27° (N = 90°); PIP = 30° (N = 100°); DIP = 24° (N = 80°)).

130. Treatment (a): If there is no significant soft-tissue injury, if the fracture is in an acceptable position, and if it is clinically and radiologically stable, treatment should be directed at controlling the initial pain and swelling. Elevation of the arm in a sling may be helpful, *provided the sling is applied in such a way that the hand is not dependent.* Any pressure dressing should avoid causing a local constriction. The finger should be mobilised early.

131. Treatment (b): If the position is unsatisfactory, the fracture should be manipulated. If a good stable position can be obtained, treat as above. If the position is acceptable, or an acceptable position has been obtained by manipulation, but the fracture is unstable, splintage will be required. For the less severe injuries buddy (garter) strapping to an adjacent finger with interdigital felt padding provides the ideal combination of stability while retaining movement.

132. Treatment (c): The injury, if severe, may require additional support by a cast or bandaging. The long-held view is that the MP joints should be flexed to 90°, the IP joints extended, and the thumb abducted (to reduce the stiffening effects of fibrosis in the collateral ligaments). In practice this position is often difficult to achieve, and Tavassoli et al[4] has shown that in metacarpal fractures short-term splintage of the MP joints in extension has no adverse effect.

133. Treatment (d): The previously described classical position for the finger joints, where return of function is expected, must be carefully differentiated from the position of *fixation* where no return of function is anticipated (e.g. the position a joint is placed in for fusion). In the latter case, the MP and IP joints are put up in mid-flexion.

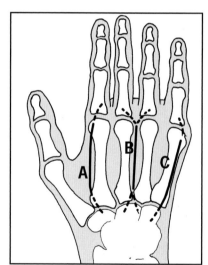

134. Treatment of unstable injuries (a): If the fracture is unstable and cannot be held with simple splintage, then the commonest and most reliable form of fixation for phalangeal (1) and metacarpal (2) fracture is by the use of Kirschner wires (within the medullary canal or using a number of other techniques). In most cases this involves closed reduction and internal fixation (CRIF) under intensifier control. They are generally left in situ until callus is visible on the radiographs.

135. Treatment for unstable injuries (b): In some cases closed reduction proves impossible, and open reduction is required. Other situations where open reduction becomes necessary include:
1. If fluoroscopy is not available.
2. If the fracture is intra-articular.
3. If the fracture is open.
4. Where there are multiple fractures in the hand. The radiograph shows an irreducible fracture of a proximal phalanx.

136. Surgical approaches (a): The metacarpals: The index metacarpal may be approached through a dorsal incision just lateral to its shaft (A); the fifth metacarpal through a dorso-lateral incision (B); and the middle, ring or both these metacarpals through an incision between them (C). The dotted lines indicate how these incisions may be extended to allow exposure of the metacarpal heads or bases.

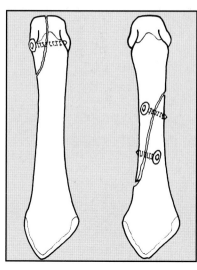

137. Surgical approaches (b): The middle and proximal phalanges: for the mid-axial approach the incision joins the ends of the skin creases revealed by flexing the finger, and is extended as required. It is developed in a slightly volar direction, at first over the mid point of the middle phalanx where there is most fat. The neurovascular bundle should be identified - it should lie 2 mm volar to the skin incision - and retracted anteriorly.

138. Surgical approaches (c): The phalanges may also be exposed through a dorsal lazy-S incision, with retraction of the extensor tendon to one side. The distal phalanx and its base may also be exposed from the dorsal aspect. An H-shaped incision may be used to create small distal and larger proximal flaps.

139. Other methods of fixation (a): Lag and other screws: These may be used to reconstruct articular fractures, or to hold unstable fractures of the metacarpals or phalanges. The bone fragments are often small and friable, and secure fixation without risk of devascularisation or fragment fracture requires careful case selection. As a general rule, any fragment should be at least three times the diameter of the screw intended to be used. (2.7 mm screws may be used in metacarpal fractures; 2.0 and 1.5 mm screws are used in phalangeal fractures.)

140. Other methods of fixation (b): Plates: These must be carefully placed to avoid interference with the gliding structures. They are of value in fractures which are comminuted (1), have bone loss, or are intra-articular or periarticular (e.g. of T- and Y- pattern) (2). Several patterns of plate are available including 1/4 tubular, DCP, and T-shaped condylar.

141. Other methods of fixation (c): Wiring techniques: The aim is to achieve a rigidity of fixation that will allow early mobilisation. The bones of the hand are small and soft tissue cover poor; and the proximity of the gliding structures add to the risks of tendon and joint adhesions. Wiring techniques are often able to address these problems.
Type A intraosseous wiring (a): This is suitable for transverse fractures, and employs a single loop of 26G monofilament stainless steel wire and a Kirschner wire.

142. Type A intraosseous wiring (b): *Technique:* The fracture may be approached through a mid-line dorsal incision (except in the case of the distal phalanx, when an H incision is used). Two transverse holes, situated marginally towards the dorsal surfaces and 3-4 mm from the bone ends, are drilled using a trocar pointed 0.035″ (0.89 mm) Kirschner wire (or equivalent drill) (1). Through these holes the wire is threaded, using if required, a 20G needle as a carrier (2). A Kirschner wire is then inserted obliquely through the distal fragment (3).

143. Type A intraosseous wiring (c): The K-wire is partially withdrawn (4), the fracture reduced, and the K-wire driven through the opposite cortex (5). The wire is twisted (6), and the ends cropped and tucked into a hole drilled in the cortex (7). External splintage (e.g. bandages, sling, POP backshell) may be used for comfort, but this should be discarded by the seventh day. A biodegradable bone peg may be used instead of the K-wire. This form of wiring is not recommended for metacarpal shaft fractures.

144. Type B intraosseous wiring: This is suitable for small articular fragments. *Technique.* The fracture is reduced, and a hole drilled at right angles to the fracture line (1). Leave the drill (0.035″ (0.89mm) K-wire) in position, and with a second drill make a hole parallel to the first (2). Insert the wire, using a hypodermic needle as a carrier, tighten, crop and bury as before (3). If the fragment is too small to drill, it may be snared by passing the wire next to bone (e.g. through the collateral ligament attachment) (4).

145. 90–90 intraosseous wiring (a): This resembles Type A wiring, but instead of a single wire (1), two wires are used at right angles to one another (2). It is a strong method of holding transverse fractures of the metacarpals and phalanges, and is useful for fusions and replants. It should not be used if there is osteoporosis or fragmentation. *Technique:* The bone ends are trimmed if necessary to provide flat contiguous surfaces, and holes drilled with careful attention to orientation.

146. 90–90 intraosseous wiring (b): A 20G needle may be used as a carrier, flexing the finger at the fracture site as required for placing the vertical wire (1 and 2). When both wires have been inserted (3), the fracture is reduced and the wires tightened by twisting. The ends should be buried to avoid interference with the gliding structures. After closure, additional external splintage may be employed for patient comfort; this should be discarded and mobilisation commenced within 7 days.

147. Tension band wiring: This can give very strong fixation, and is useful for unstable fractures of the phalanges and metacarpals, especially when there is a degree of fragmentation. *Technique.* The fractures are reduced and held with single or paired Kirschner wires; the wires are cropped so that the amount protruding from the bone is just enough to give anchorage for tension band wires. These are looped round the *dorsal* surface of the bone before tightening.

148. Rigid mini external fixators (d): Small external fixators may be used for multifragmentary fractures, fractures with bone loss and/or severe soft-tissue involvement, infected fractures, and fracture dislocations of the PIP joint. Traction (e.g. for joint disruptions) or compression techniques may be employed. Unilateral, bilateral, and combination systems (Illus.) can be used. Their application can be difficult, the pin tracks are susceptible to infection, and the pins may interfere with the gliding structures.

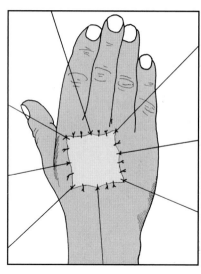

149. Motion permitting external fixators (e): The Compass PIP Joint Hinge®, centred over the axis of movement of the joint, is attached to two pins on either side of the fracture, controlling the position of the fragments as in other external fixators, and permitting a degree of distraction to encourage alignment of fragments (particularly intra-articular ones). The worm may be disengaged to permit active movements, or it may be engaged and advanced for passive mobilisation.

150. Soft-tissue management (a): Where there is necrotic or foreign material, a thorough debridement should be performed under a tourniquet to minimise the risks of infection. There is little tissue to spare in the hand, and wide excision of wounds is to be avoided. The tourniquet should be released prior to closure to secure bleeding points and reduce wound haematoma.

151. Soft-tissue management (b): Where there is skin loss, every attempt should be made to ensure that healing will be achieved as quickly as possible to permit early mobilisation. The exposure of fractures, joints and bones should be avoided, and if the situation permits a primary skin grafting procedure or plastic repair should be carried out.

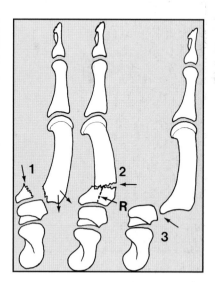

152. Soft-tissue management (c): If there is division of both neurovascular bundles to a finger, amputation should be advised unless facilities for microsurgery are available and the particular circumstances (e.g. employment, hobbies, etc.) make an attempt at preservation particularly desirable. In all cases, the maximum length of thumb must be preserved.

153. Soft-tissue management (d): If there is appreciable risk of infection (e.g. ragged wound, dirty causal instrument) primary suture of nerves and also of tendons in the 'no man's area' of the tendon sheaths should not be undertaken. Where, however, the circumstances are ideal the experienced surgeon may achieve the best results by primary repair.

154. Injuries to the thumb: The base: The commonest injuries involving the base of the thumb are (1) Bennett's fracture (or Bennett's fracture-dislocation as it may be more aptly called); (2) fractures of the base of the thumb metacarpal. When there is a vertical extension into the joint, converting it into a T- or Y-fracture, the prognosis is less good (Rolando fracture); (3) carpometacarpal dislocation of the thumb.

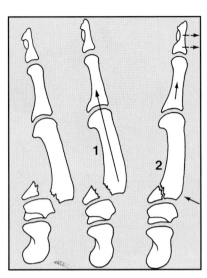

155. Diagnosis: Injuries of the base usually result from force being applied along the long axis of the thumb – e.g. from a fall or blow on the clenched fist (1) – or from forced abduction of the thumb (2). Any of these may be mistaken for scaphoid fracture, but tenderness is maximal distal to the snuff box (and deformity may be obvious).

156. Bennett's fracture: Note the distinctive features of this fracture: 1. a small medial fragment of bone which may tilt, but maintains its relationship with the trapezium, 2. the (vertical) fracture line involves the joint between the thumb metacarpal and the trapezium (trapezometacarpal joint), 3. most important, the proximal and lateral subluxation of the thumb metacarpal.

157. Treatment (a): The principle of reduction is straightforward: traction is applied to the thumb (1) and reduction completed by abducting it and applying pressure to the lateral aspect of the base (2). A general anaesthetic or Bier block is usually necessary. Maintaining reduction can be troublesome, but this may be achieved by either internal fixation or a carefully applied plaster cast.

158. Treatment (b): After reduction, subsequent subluxation of the metacarpal may be prevented and the fracture held by (1) screw fixation (e.g. using the AO small fragment set, with further stabilisation of the fixation with a Kirschner wire); or (2) the use of two Kirschner wires.

159. Treatment (c): Cast fixation (i): Alternatively, plaster fixation may be used provided attention is paid to the details. (a) Begin by applying stockingette to the arm (1) and the thumb (2). Bony prominences should be protected as required with wool roll (3). (b) A small felt pad is placed over the base of the thumb metacarpal (4). (*Note:* adhesive felt should not be applied directly to the skin in this situation if a pustular rash is to be avoided.)

160. Cast fixation (ii): An assistant applies traction to the thumb and steadies the lateral three fingers (1). (d) Two to three 15 cm (6″) POP bandages (with or without an anterior slab) are applied to the *forearm* (2). (e) Two 10 cm (4″) POP bandages are then quickly applied to the wrist and up to the IP joint of the thumb (3).

161. Cast fixation (iii): The surgeon now takes the thumb (the plaster being set on the forearm while the distal part remains soft). He must apply traction (1), abduct the thumb (2), maintain pressure over the base of the first metacarpal (3), and mould the plaster well into the MP joint on its flexor aspect (4).

162. Cast fixation (iv): Aftercare:
1. Check radiographs are taken to confirm that reduction has been achieved.
2. The arm may require elevating with a sling for the first few days.
3. The patient should be seen at weekly intervals for the first 2-3 weeks and the thumb X-rayed. If the plaster appears slack at any stage it must be changed. If there is evidence of slipping of the fracture a new plaster should also be applied (no anaesthetic is generally required). During the setting of the plaster, light traction should be applied to the thumb while the plaster is well moulded round the base (in the position described for the initial reduction).
4. Plaster fixation should be maintained for 6 weeks.

Cullen and others[5] suggest that provided the thumb metacarpal is aligned with the trapezium and the metacarpal fragment, a fracture gap of up to 2 mm need not cause concern, and is unlikely to lead to secondary osteoarthritis.

163. Fractures near the base of the thumb metacarpal: Greenstick fractures of this type are common in children. Angulation is usually slight or moderate, and should be accepted; gross angulations should be manipulated, using the technique described for Bennett's fracture. Plaster fixation for about 5 weeks is desirable. **Rolando fractures** require careful reduction, and good results are claimed for stabilisation with an external fixator, the pins being placed in the metacarpal and the trapezium.

164. Carpometacarpal dislocation of the thumb: The thumb may dislocate at the joint between the metacarpal base and the traezium, or the whole of the first ray may be involved, the trapezium remaining with the thumb metacarpal, with the dislocation taking place between the trapezium and the scaphoid (Illus.). Both these injuries result from forcible abduction of the thumb. *Treatment:* Reduce by applying traction to thumb and local pressure over the base. Any persisting instability may be controlled with percutaneous K-wires. Thereafter apply a well-padded plaster of scaphoid type for 3 weeks. Elevation of the limb for the first few days is desirable. Physiotherapy is seldom required.

165. Injuries at the MP joint of the thumb: Posterior dislocation (a): This injury generally results from forcible hyperextension of the thumb. It is common in children. In a number of cases there is 'button holing' of the capsule by the metacarpal head and closed methods of reduction will fail. Nevertheless, manipulation should be tried first in all cases.

166. Posterior dislocation (b): Manipulative reduction may often be attempted without anaesthesia (by the quick confident application of the traction to the thumb with simultaneous pressure over the metacarpal head). When open reduction is required this should be performed through a lateral incision under a tourniquet. In all cases a light plaster splint should be worn for 2-3 weeks after reduction.

167. Rupture of the ulnar collateral ligament (Gamekeeper's thumb) (a): This injury is caused by forcible abduction (1). If unrecognised and untreated, there may be progressive MP subluxation (2) with interference with grasp, causing significant permanent disability. *Suspect* this injury when there is complaint of pain in this region. *Look for tenderness* on the medial side of the MP joint.

168. Ulnar collateral ligament (b): Extend the MP joint fully and apply stress to the ulnar collateral ligament by abducting the proximal phalanx. Repeat with the thumb flexed at the MP joint. Note the presence of any 'give'. Carefully compare one side with the other. If in doubt, stress radiographs should be taken. Careful palpation may reveal the torn distal portion of the ligament lodged between the adductor pollicis aponeurosis and its normal position (Stener lesion).

169. Ulnar collateral ligament (c): Study radiographs of the joint: 1. Subluxation may or may not be apparent in the unstressed films. 2. An avulsion fracture (Illus.) may betray this type of injury (sometimes separately referred to as gamekeeper's fracture). If a fracture is present, note its position. (Marked displacement, or rotation so that its articular surface is pointing distally and a large fragment are indications for surgery.)

170. Ulnar collateral ligament (d): *Treatment:* 1. Slight laxity or minimally displaced avulsion fracture: scaphoid cast for 6 weeks (1); 2. Rotated fragment: reduction and internal fixation; 3. Gross laxity, especially with a palpable Stener lesion: primary surgical repair is usually preferred. (Conservative treatment may give a good result but is less reliable.) 4. Late diagnosed complete tear: repair of the capsulo-ligamentous complex with a palmaris longus free tendon graft; or as a salvage procedure, MP joint fusion (2).

171. Fracture of the proximal phalanx: The severely angled fracture (1) should be reduced by traction and local pressure. Hold with a dorsal (or volar) slab (2) to which is added a girdered extension (3), held on with bandages. If the position cannot be readily held, internal fixation (e.g. by one of the wiring methods) is indicated. The minimally angled fracture (4) or the splinter fracture (5) may be protected by a local slab (similar to 3) bandaged in position. Elevation may be required.

172. IP joint dislocation of the thumb: Reduce by traction as described for MP joint dislocations. Only occasionally is anaesthesia required (ring or Bier block). Thereafter splint for 2-3 weeks with a local plaster slab. *Fractures of the terminal phalanx:* Crushing injuries are the usual cause, and any soft-tissue damage takes priority in management. A light local splint (e.g. of plaster) will prevent pain from stubbing.

173. Injuries to the fifth metacarpal: The commonest fractures involving the metacarpal of the little finger are: (1) fractures of the neck, (2) spiral fractures of the shaft, usually undisplaced (3) transverse fractures of the shaft, often angulated, (4) fractures of the base, (5) fractures of the head. (b = base, h = head.)

174. Fractures of the neck of the fifth metacarpal (a): These are nearly always caused by the clenched fist meeting resistance, for example, as a result of a fight (1). Angulation and impaction are common (2). When angulation is slight (3) or moderate (4) it should be accepted, and the fracture supported for 3-4 weeks until local pain settles.

175. Neck of fifth metacarpal (b): A simple dorsal slab (1), completed after a few days, may be quite satisfactory. Better fixation is achieved by the addition of a finger extension (2) to the basic slab. Still more support is provided by the use of buddy (garter) strapping (3) and the inclusion of the ring and little fingers in the extension (4) (securing bandages omitted in Illus. for clarity).

176. Neck of fifth metacarpal (c): If angulation is gross (more than 45°), an attempt may be made to correct it. The MP joint is flexed; pressure is then applied to the head via the proximal phalanx, using the thumb. The fingers apply counter-pressure to the shaft. Reduction is generally easy. The position may be maintained using a Kirschner wire or with a plaster cast.

177. Neck of fifth metacarpal (d): The following technique may be employed. Stockingette is applied to the arm (1) and to the little finger (2). A thin strip of felt (3) is placed over the finger (4). A substantial dorsal slab is applied (5). The finger should be flexed into the palm and the striking point checked (see Frame 127).

178. Neck of fifth metacarpal (e): A finger slab, made from a thrice-folded slab formed from three layers or so of 10 cm (4″) plaster bandage (6) is applied from wrist to fingertip (7). Pressure is maintained while the slab is setting. Meanwhile an assistant can be securing the slabs with a wet gauze bandage (8). Complete in 2-3 days and retain for 3 weeks only.

179. Injuries of the fifth metacarpal *ctd:* Spiral fractures of the shaft (2), transverse fractures of the shaft with slight or moderate angulation or displacement (3) and fractures of the base (4) may be treated quite adequately by the application of a Colles plaster for 3-4 weeks.

180. Injuries of the fifth metacarpal *ctd:* Marked angulation of a shaft fracture should be treated by traction and local pressure prior to plaster fixation (1). Displaced fractures may be similarly reduced (2); if unstable they may be held with 1-2 intramedullary K-wires inserted through the neck of the metatarsal. Soft tissue between the bone ends may necessitate open reduction, when the position may be maintained by percutaneous (3) or intramedullary Kirschner wiring, 90-90 intraosseous wiring, or plating.

181. Injuries of the fifth metacarpal *ctd:* Fractures of the *head* of the fifth metacarpal (see 5, Frame 173) may be treated by buddy strapping and early mobilisation; if symptoms are marked a dorsal slab may also be used for the first 1-2 weeks. If the fragment is substantial and displaced, internal fixation using a screw or Type B intraosseous wiring may be considered. *Dislocation of the base* of the metacarpal (Illus.) is usually easily reduced with traction, but may need Kirschner wire stabilisation.

182. Injuries to the middle and ring metatarsals: The so-called *inboard fractures* involving the third and fourth metacarpals are inherently stable as they are attached by muscle and ligament to one another and to the stable pillars formed by second and fifth metacarpals. The commonest fracture is a spiral or transverse fracture of the shaft, especially the fourth metacarpal, but fractures involving both or of the base and neck are frequent. Undisplaced fractures may be supported by a Colles type slab, but be on guard for swelling which can be severe, especially in multiple fractures.

When the AP radiographs show the presence of an isolated off-ended fracture (i.e. where there is complete loss of bony apposition) affecting the middle or ring metacarpals, or where there is moderate angulation or shortening, the position can generally be accepted. The striking point of the finger, however, should be checked, a dorsal slab applied and the limb elevated to counteract swelling. If off-ending or angulation is conspicuous in the *lateral projection*, reduction should be carried out, either by manipulation or by an open procedure.

183. Injuries to the index metacarpal: The so-called *outboard fractures* involve the second and fifth metacarpals. Fractures of the fifth metacarpal have already been dealt with and severely displaced fractures of the index should be managed along similar lines. In particular, badly displaced fractures should be reduced, and if necessary secured by some form of internal fixation. If Kirschner wires are used they should be retained for 3 weeks; plaster fixation may be needed for a further 2 weeks.

184. Fractures of the proximal and middle phalanges: Undisplaced, simple fractures, e.g. of the shaft (1), base (2), neck (3), intercondylar region (4) or epiphyseal injuries (5), seldom present any problem. Buddy strapping (6) for 3–4 weeks may give adequate support, but if symptoms are marked this may be supplemented by the use of a volar or dorsal slab, with finger extension. Displaced fractures should be assessed and treated as previously indicated (Frame 125 et seq.).

185. Aftercare: In all cases: 1. uninjured fingers should be left free and exercised, 2. rigid fixation should be discarded as soon as possible. In many situations where a cast support has been used initially, buddy (garter) strapping may be substituted after 2 weeks, and often all support after 4.

Complications: Finger stiffness is the commonest and most disabling complication, and is due to joint adhesions, fibrosis in the adjacent flexor tendon sheaths and collateral ligament shortening. Infection in open fractures may be a major contributory factor. Stiffness may be minimised by the procedures described (e.g. elevation, correct splinting, early mobilisation) and by intensive physiotherapy and occupational therapy. Physiotherapy and occupational therapy should be continued with vigour until the range of movements and finger power become static. This implies careful recording, at frequent intervals, of these parameters. In this respect it is helpful to note the *total active range of motion* (TAM) in each digit; this overall movement can be assessed by a single goniometer measurement; it is a little less than the sum of the normal maxima of flexion of the individual joints, the normal value of TAM being taken to be 250°.

Early return to work should be encouraged to foster adaptation. Inability to work and a static response to physiotherapy require a most careful assessment of the following: 1. possibility of redeployment, 2. possibility of improvement from further surgery (e.g. tenolysis), 3. amputation.

Amputation as primary treatment must be raised in open phalangeal fractures when they are associated with flexor tendon division. Division of one or both neurovascular bundles, skin loss or severe crushing are additional factors weighing in favour of this procedure (in contrast to attempted repair where treatment is likely to be prolonged and the final result uncertain). With these factors must be considered the patient's age, sex and occupation.

Mal-union: Problems may arise from: (i) recurrence of deformity, (ii) failure to correct initial deformity, (iii) torsional deformity. In some cases (iv) epiphyseal displacement may have escaped attention. In the latter case remodelling may lead to correction, and in the others trick movements and postural adaptations may remove the patient's initial strong desire for corrective surgery. It is wise not to offer surgical correction until at least 6 months have passed since the injury.

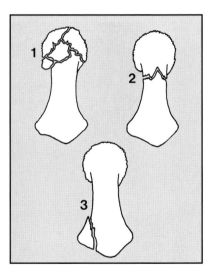

186. Fractures of the terminal phalanx: Fractures of the terminal tuft (often comminuted) (1), of the neck (2), and the base (3) are painful but relatively unimportant injuries. Treatment of any associated soft tissue injury takes precedence (e.g. debridement and suture of pulp lacerations). Nevertheless, strapping the finger to a spatula or use of a plastic finger splint may relieve pain and prevent any painful stubbing incidents.

187. Mallet finger (a): This is caused by forcible flexion of an extended finger. The distal extensor tendon slip is torn at its attachment to bone (Type I injury) or avulses a fragment of bone (Type II). The patient is unable to extend the DIP joint fully; drooping of the fingertip may be slight (a) or severe (b). In late cases there may be hyperextension of the PIP joint (c). In Type III injuries, more than 20% of the articular surface of the distal phalanx is involved, sometimes with anterior subluxation of the phalanx.

188. Mallet finger (b): *Treatment:* All these injuries excepting Type IIIs with subluxation may be treated by splinting the distal joint in extension. A Stack or Abuna splint (Illus.) may be used. Choose the size with care to lessen the risks of skin ulceration. It is strapped to the finger and worn for 6 weeks constantly, and then for a further 2 at night only. It may be removed for skin hygiene if extension is preserved. Alternatively, support the distal joint with a short length of padded spatula strapped to the volar surface.

189. Mallet finger (c): Where the patient's cooperation is in doubt, a Smillie plaster may be used for 6–8 weeks, although it can cause some stiffness. Form a 4-layer tube of 7.5 cm (3″) dry POP bandage round the finger. Dip the hand momentarily in water, asking the patient to flex the PIP joint and extend the DIP joint against the thumb while the POP is smoothed. *Note:* In any case there may be some recurrence on removal of splintage, but disability is seldom more than slight, and spontaneous improvement may occur up to a year after the injury.

190. Mallet finger (d): If there is subluxation, splint in flexion or extension if reduction can be achieved in that position: otherwise repair is advised through a C-shaped incision. A pull-out wire may be used with a stabilising K-wire as illustrated, but a suture anchor (such as the Mitek® Micro QuickAnchor®) may be preferred. *Late diagnosed:* Extension splintage may be successful even as late as 6 months. If there is a swan-neck deformity, an oblique retinacular ligament reconstruction has been advocated.

191. MP and interphalangeal joint dislocations: These may be simple or multiple (Illus.) and as they result from hyperextension are almost always posterior dislocations. Reduce as described for the thumb (Frame 165). Thereafter buddy strapping should be applied for 2 weeks unless there is any evidence of instability – when plaster of Paris splintage may be required for a slightly longer period.

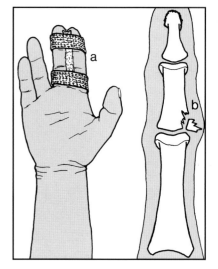

192. Fracture dislocation: It is essential that the joint surface is correctly relocated, and important that mobilisation is commenced as soon as possible. Open reduction is usually required, and fixation may be achieved with intraosseous wiring, small fragment set screws, or plating; in some cases a motion permitting external fixator may be used. Mobilisation should be commenced immediately with the added support of buddy strapping.

193. 'Sprains' and lateral subluxations (a): These are usually caused by falls in which the side of a finger strikes some resistant object. There is avulsion or tearing of a collateral ligament. Spontaneous reduction is the rule. *Diagnosis:* The injury should be suspected on the basis of the history and the presence of local tenderness. Confirmation is obtained by noting instability on stressing the collateral ligament.

194. Sprains and lateral subluxations (b): Radiographs may show a tell-tale avulsion fracture. If doubt remains, stress films may be taken. Treatment: (a) Buddy strapping for 5 weeks should be adequate. (b) If an avulsion fracture is present and has rotated, it should be replaced and fixed. *Complications:* Fusiform swellings of the finger may persist for many months even in the treated injury. If a flexion deformity starts to develop, use an extension assisting lively splint.

195. Compartment syndromes in the hand: There are no less than 10 osteofascial compartments in the hand (7 for the interossei, 1 thenar, 1 hypothenar, and 1 containing adductor pollicis). Increased compartment pressure may follow severe crushing injuries, multiple fractures, and the erroneous administration of unsuitable intravenous infusions. The onset may be heralded by severe pain, loss of finger movements, and increased swelling. The fingers are usually held in a position of extension at the MP joints, and flexion at the proximal IP joints. Sensory disturbance is not a feature.

The increased tissue pressure required to produce this condition is about 10 mm lower than that found at other sites.

Treatment: The transverse carpal ligament must be divided. If a midline incision is used then access to the three anterior compartments may be readily obtained through it.

The interosseous compartments may be opened through two longitudinal dorsal incisions (over the second and fourth metacarpals). The dorsal incisions may be closed primarily, but secondary closure is usually advised for the volar incision.

196. AO Classification of fractures of the radius/ulna, distal segment (23–):

Type A fractures are extra-articular.
A1 = Fracture of the ulna only: .1 styloid process; .2 simple, of the metaphysis; .3 multifragmentary of the metaphysis.
A2 = Simple impacted fracture of the radius: .1 undisplaced; .2 with dorsal tilting (Colles pattern); .3 with anterior tilting (Smith pattern).
A3 = Multifragmentary fracture of the radius: .1 with axial impaction and shortening; .2 with a wedge; .3 complex.

Type B fractures are partial articular fractures of the radius.
B1 = Partial articular fracture of radius in the sagittal plane: .1 simple lateral; .2 multifragmentary lateral; .3 medial.
B2 = Partial articular fracture of the radius with involvement of the posterior lip (dorsal rim) (Barton's fracture): .1 simple; .2 with an additional lateral sagittal fracture; .3 with dorsal dislocation of the carpus (fracture dislocation of the wrist).
B3 = Partial articular fracture of the radius with involvement of the anterior lip (volar rim) (Reverse Barton's fracture): .1 simple with a small fragment; .2 simple with a large fragment; .3 multifragmentary.

Type C fractures are complete articular fractures.
C1 = Both the metaphyseal and articular elements are simple; .1 with a posteromedial articular fragment; .2 with the articular fracture line in the sagittal plane; .3 with articular fracture line in the frontal plane.
C2 = The articular fracture is simple, but the metaphyseal fracture is multifragmentary: .1 the articular fracture line is in the sagittal plane; .2 the articular fracture line is in the frontal plane; .3 the metaphyseal fracture extends into the diaphysis.
C3 = The articular fracture is multifragmentary: .1 metaphyseal simple; .2 the metaphyseal fracture is also multifragmentary; .3 multifragmentary metaphyseal fracture extending into the diaphysis.

19. Dermatomes (a): In the upper limb, the anterior axial line follows the line of the second rib from the angle of Louis, and continues down the anterior aspect of the arm, splitting near the middle finger which is supplied by C7. The other dermatomes are arranged in a regular fashion on either side of the axial line. If indicated, a **sensory index score** may be made for each limb (0 = absent sensation; 1 = impaired; 2 = normal).

20. Dermatomes (b): The lumbar and sacral dermatomes have a complex arrangement which is difficult to commit to memory. Remember by the facts that: 1. The outer border of the foot is supplied by S1; 2. The medial part of the foot and the lateral part of the leg by L5; 3. The 'stocking top' area is supplied by L2 and 4. the saddle area by S3. 'We kneel on L3, stand on S1, and sit on S3.'

21. DETERMINING THE SEVERITY OF NEUROLOGICAL INVOLVEMENT

It is helpful to record the extent of any neurological impairment, and the Frankel Scale is a simple and direct method of doing so:

Frankel A: complete paralysis
Frankel B: only sensory function below the injury level
Frankel C: incomplete motor function below the injury level
Frankel D: fair to good motor function below the injury level
Frankel E: normal function

TYPES OF INCOMPLETE CORD INJURY:

A number of cord syndromes are recognised. These include the following.

Anterior column syndrome The damage is to the anterior two thirds of the cord and commonly occurs in burst fractures of the spine where there is compression of the cord and interruption of its blood supply by fragments of bone which have been forced into the spinal canal. There is complete motor paralysis and loss of sensation to pin prick and light touch, but proprioception and perception of deep pressure are retained. There is greater muscle loss in the legs than in the arms. This has the worst prognosis of all cord syndromes, with only 10–15% having any functional recovery. No return of sensation to pin prick or temperature in the sacral area after 24 hours is a very poor prognostic indicator.

Central cord syndrome This is the commonest incomplete cord syndrome, and generally follows a hyperextension injury. It is particularly common in the older patient who has a degree of cervical spondylosis (see also Frame 71). The cord may be affected over several segments, with involvement of both grey and white matter. The effects are curiously greater in the arms than in the legs. In the upper limbs, lower motor neurone lesions predominate, with a partial flaccid paralysis of the fingers and arms, and loss of pain and temperature sensation. In the lower limbs the lesion is an upper motor one, resulting in a spastic paralysis, usually with sparing of sensation, but sometimes with bladder and bowel involvement. This lesion pattern is sometimes referred to as 'man in a barrel' syndrome (MIB), a typical example being an elderly man who is able to walk but whose shoulders are immobile and his hands anaesthetic.

Brown-Séquard syndrome This most commonly results from a unilateral facet joint fracture or dislocation and is due to hemitransection or similar damage to the cord. There is muscle paralysis and loss of discriminatory and joint sensation on the side of the injury, and loss of pain and temperature sensation on the other. The syndrome has a good prognosis, with more than 90% regaining bowel and bladder control and the ability to walk.

Posterior cord syndrome Injuries to the posterior cord are rare, but may follow injuries associated with rupture of the posterior ligament complex or penetrating wounds. There is loss of vibration and position sense, but motor function and pain and temperature sensation are retained.

Cauda equina syndrome Urinary retention is the most consistent finding (see p. 268) and partial injuries often have a good prognosis. In any suspected lesion examine for saddle anaesthesia, rectal tone, the bulbocavernosus reflex and sacral sparing.

THE COMMON LESIONS

1. Spinal concussion causes a temporary arrest of conduction within the cord; its effects are patchy and recovery is rapid. If, for example, there is a *complete* spinal lesion on first examination, spinal concussion is an unlikely but possible cause. If after 12 hours the lesion remains complete, spinal concussion is *not* the cause.
2. If there is any evidence of voluntary motor activity, skin sensation or proprioception below the level of the lesion, the cord has not been transected (and further recovery is possible).
3. After an injury to the cord, the reflexes generally disappear for at least some hours, and sometimes for as long as 2 weeks. Return of reflex activity with continued absence of all sensation and voluntary muscle contraction confirms a *transection of the cord*.
4. Where the injury is at a level where there is potential damage to lumbar nerve roots or the cauda equina (e.g. injuries at the thoracolumbar junction) persistent absence of reflexes would confirm such damage.
5. Note that cord transection is irrecoverable, but there is potential recovery where there is involvement of nerve roots and the cauda equina.

22. Injuries to the cervical spine:
Diagnosis: Suspect involvement of the cervical spine where the patient: 1. Complains of neck, occipital or shoulder pain after trauma; 2. Has a torticollis (Illus.), complains of restriction of neck movements or supports the head with the hands, or 3. Is found unconscious after a head injury, especially in road traffic accidents. In all cases, further investigation by radiographs is essential.

23. Initial management (a): If you suspect that the cervical spine has been injured, your first move should be to safeguard the cord by controlling neck movements. The simplest and best way of doing this is by applying a cervical collar. (Illus.: commercially available collar adjustable in depth and girth.) At the roadside, an adequate collar may be fashioned from rolled newspapers pushed into a nylon stocking and wrapped round the neck.

24. Initial management (b): Alternatively, if the patient is on a trolley, the head may be supported by sandbags. *Do not allow the head to flex forwards, and do not hyperextend.* Keep the head in a neutral position wherever possible, and in the conscious patient quickly check that there is active movement in all limbs.

27. Initial management (e): Investigate further if there is persistent limitation of movements or evidence of neurological disturbance. CT and MRI scans are likely to provide the best additional information. *CT scans* may help show hard-to-see fractures, especially of the neural arches and facet joints, and define any neural canal encroachment in burst fractures.

    MRI scans may be able to show the state of the posterior ligament complex and the intervertebral discs. Alternatively, the following additional radiographs should be taken: 1. Two more lateral projections, one in flexion and one in extension; these again should be supervised; 2. Right and left oblique projections of the cervical spine.

    The commonest difficulty is the technical one of visualising the lower cervical vertebrae in the stocky patient. The upper border of T1 *must* be seen. *Accept* that detail may be poor. *Do not accept* that the spine cannot be shown in sufficient detail to exclude dislocation of one vertebra over another. If necessary, assist the radiographer by arranging for traction to be applied to the arms – one in adduction and the other in abduction; slight angulation of the tube and increase in exposure may be helpful. In some cases screening of the cervical spine movements may be useful.

25. Initial management (c): Especially if there is some evidence of neurological involvement, *do not* check the range of movements in the cervical spine. Accompany the patient to the X-ray department, supporting the head during the positioning of the tube and making sure that the spine is not forced in to flexion. For initial screening an AP, lateral and a through-the-mouth projection of C1 and C2 should be taken.

26. Initial management (d): If these films appear normal, you may proceed in reasonable safety to 1. Further examination of the neck for localising tenderness, restriction of active movements and protective spasm, and 2. A more thorough neurological examination. If these show no departure from normal, the patient may be treated with a cervical collar, with a follow-up review in 1 week.

28. Classification of cervical spine injuries: Injuries of the cervical spine may be grouped according to the mechanism of injury:
(1) Flexion (anterior compression) injuries
(2) Flexion and rotation injuries
(3) Extension injuries
(4) Burst (vertical compression) fractures.
(Note that injuries involving the *proximal* cervical spine are dealt with separately at the end of the following section.)

29. Causes of flexion and flexion/rotation injuries: These may result from: 1. Falls on the back of the head leading to flexion of the neck, e.g. in motor cycle spills, diving in shallow water, pole vaulting and rugby football. 2. Blows on the back of the head from falling objects (e.g. in the building and mining industries). 3. Rapid deceleration in head-on car accidents.

30. Flexion injuries: Stable anterior wedge (compression) fracture (a): The vertebral body is wedged anteriorly, while the posterior part is generally intact. Instability *must* be excluded: there must be no evidence of injury to the posterior ligament complex, with no separation of the vertebral spines (which the radiograph here suggests may possibly be present). Check if possible with an MRI scan. Eliminate damage to the neural arches or facets. Flexion and extension laterals may be carried out to exclude instability.

31. Stable anterior wedge fracture (b): Assuming these criteria are satisfied, neurological disturbance is rare and the prognosis excellent. Treat with a cervical collar for 6 weeks. Rarely when there is a degree of lateral wedging there may be troublesome nerve root involvement usually with (mainly) sensory disturbance in the corresponding dermatome. *If instability is at all suspected, treat as a cervical dislocation.*

32. Flexion/rotation injuries: Unilateral dislocation with a locked facet joint (a): One facet joint dislocates, so that in the lateral projection of the cervical spine one vertebral body is seen to overlap the one below (i.e. there is anterior translation of the upper vertebra with regard to the vertebra below) by about a third. The AP view may not be helpful, or it may show malalignment of spinous processes. There is often little difference between laterals taken in flexion and extension.

33. Unilateral dislocation (b): Oblique projections will, however, confirm the diagnosis. On one side the columnar arrangement of bodies, foramina and facet joints will be regular (Illus.), while on the other (see next frame) it will be broken. Damage to the posterior ligament complex is variable, and *after reduction* these injuries may be quite stable – **but note:** if there is an associated fracture involving a facet joint the injury is **most certainly unstable** and after reduction, fusion will be required.

34. Unilateral dislocation (c): The oblique radiograph shows a dislocated facet joint. In all cases requiring reduction a pre-operative MRI scan should be carried out to exclude a disc rupture: a significant prolapse may merit an anterior discectomy and interbody fusion in case manipulation precipitates a further disc protrusion and a catastrophic neurological problem. In the elderly especially, manipulative reduction also carries a risk of causing a central cord syndrome, so that an open procedure may then be preferred.

35. Unilateral dislocation (d): On clinical examination of the patient with a unilateral dislocation, the head is slightly rotated and inclined to the side (1) away from the locked facet (2). There is often great pain with radiation (3) due to pressure on the nerve root at the level of the affected joint, and (rarely) there may be cord involvement. Proceed to treatment if there is no neurological defect or significant disc prolapse: *otherwise see* Frame 25.

36. Treatment (a): The initial aim in treatment is to reduce the dislocation, and the secret of this is well-controlled traction. 1. The patient is given a general anaesthetic; the head must be well supported during induction, the administration of any muscle relaxant and intubation (which must be carried out without undue extension of the neck). 2. X-ray facilities should be available (preferably an image intensifier).

37. Treatment (b): 3.The surgeon must have freedom to manipulate the head, and may do this with the patient fully on the table, or pulled up till the head is supported in the lap of the surgeon seated at the top end of the table. Place the thumbs under the jaw, clasp the fingers behind the occiput, and apply firm traction in *lateral flexion* away from the side of the locked facet, i.e. in the direction the head is usually inclined.

38. Treatment (c): 4. Maintaining traction, bring the head into the midline position, correcting the rotation element *before* lateral flexion. Release the traction, support the head (e.g. with foam plastic blocks) and confirm reduction with the image intensifier or by check radiographs. If, however, reduction has not been achieved, repeat the manoeuvre with greater anaesthetic relaxation. If reduction fails (rare), or if preferred, apply traction using skull tongs or a halo as for a bilateral facet dislocation.

39. Treatment (d): 5. Once reduction has been achieved, a cervical collar should be applied, and worn continuously for 6 weeks. 6. Fortnightly radiographs of the neck should be taken, and flexion and extension laterals at the end of the 6 weeks' fixation. *If there is any evidence of late subluxation* (Illus.) the patient should be admitted for a segmental posterior cervical fusion with internal fixation. Some also advocate fusion if the initial displacement is more than 25% or 3.5mm.

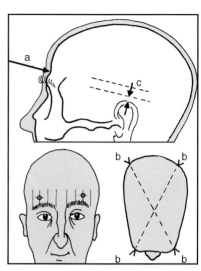

40. Flexion/rotation injuries: Unstable injuries (a): The commonest injury is a *cervical dislocation without fracture.* Displacement may be severe, and there is frequently locking of both facets. Damage to the posterior ligament complex is always present. (This may be associated with an avulsion fracture of a spinous process, widening of the gap between two spinous processes or *evidence of forward slip on a flexion lateral.*) An MRI scan is advised to exclude a significant disc prolapse. (See Frame 70.)

41. Unstable injuries (b): Skull traction will be required to achieve and maintain reduction and should be applied without delay. This may be carried out using a halo (which at a later stage may be attached to a vest or plaster jacket for continued support). The Bremer range includes (a) adjustable rings; (b) halo-crown devices; (c) small, large and custom built paediatric rings; (d) traction hoops. (Note that where there is no fracture, fusion will be required.)

42. Halo traction pin sites: Palpate the groove (a) between the superciliary ridge and the frontal prominence: the anterior pins should lie on this line, caudal to the maximal circumference of the skull, and about 1 cm above the orbital margin. Each should lie in the line of the outer half of the eyebrow (e.g. at the junction of the middle and outer thirds). The posterior pins should be sited diagonally opposite (b), at such a level that the halo band clears the ear by about a half centimetre (c). (Note that the use of 6 pins is said to reduce the risks of complications.)

43. Halo application *ctd:* Support the head manually throughout the procedure. The head of the supine patient should be just clear of the bed, with a board between the shoulder blades extending up to the occiput. Shave and prep the skin round the areas of the proposed pin sites. Slide the halo into position, and hold it with 3–4 suction cups screwed into the halo (a), positioned away from the skull pin sites. These may then be infiltrated (through the holes in the halo) with local anaesthetic (b).

44. Halo application *ctd:* Adjust the suction cups to ensure the halo is centred. Using the fingers at first, screw in opposite pairs of skull pins, before repeating this with the other pair. (At this stage some make small skin incisions to avoid indentation of the skin.) Now tighten them in stages – again in a diametrically opposed sequence – to a maximum torque of 8 inch/pounds (0.90 Newton/metre), using a torque wrench or torque limiting caps. Then attach a traction hoop. (See Frame 58 for after care.)

45. Applying skull tongs (a): Alternatively, skull tongs may be used when no later need for a halo-vest is anticipated. Several types of calliper are available, and the following description applies to those of Cone's pattern. Shave the skin round the proposed insertion points (approximately 6–7 cm above the external auditory meati) and infiltrate the areas deeply on both sides with local anaesthetic.

46. Applying skull tongs (b): Make a small incision (about 1 cm in length) on each side down to bone (b). Bleeding is usually brisk, but generally controllable by firm local pressure applied for a few moments; if not, secure and tie off any remaining bleeding points. Now insinuate one point holder through the temporalis muscle fibres until it is in contact with the skull (c).

47. Applying skull tongs (c): Keep the point holder pressed firmly against the skull; straighten out the calliper, and close it with the turnbuckle spanner (d). Guide the second point holder through the skin wound; oscillate the calliper slightly to allow its tapered end to part the temporalis fibres on the second side (e). Close the calliper until both point holders are in firm but not hard contact with the skull.

48. Applying skull tongs (d): Now screw the points in (you should check that their protrusion is limited to about 3 mm) to penetrate the outer cortex only (f); tighten them with a key. If the points fail to enter, either they are blunt or the bone unduly hard. In these circumstances, a small awl may be used as a starter, taking great care to avoid penetration of the inner cortex. Now seal the wound with strips of gauze soaked in Nobecutane™ or a similar preparation.

49. Other traction devices: *Blackburn callipers* (2) are designed to hook into the diploë of the skull, and a trephine is used to remove a tiny lid of outer cortex. Occasionally no diploë is present, and the points must hook under the full thickness of the skull, and come in contact with the dura. *Crutchfield traction tongs* (3) are inserted nearer the vertex than the other two devices.

50. Reduction (a): Assuming there is no disc prolapse (which might precipitate a neurological problem – see Frame 70), many surgeons prefer to carry out a manual reduction. General anaesthesia with good relaxation and X-ray facilities are essential. Great care must be taken during induction and throughout to avoid uncontrolled movements of the head. When all is ready, the head is supported and the end of the table dropped; firm traction is applied in the neutral position or slight flexion (1) to unlock the facets (2).

51. Reduction (b): Maintaining firm traction the neck is slowly extended (3). The hand supporting the occiput may be moved in anticipation down the neck to act as a fulcrum (4). The traction is then slowly reduced, the table end raised and, whilst maintaining a little controlling traction, the position is checked with radiographs.

52. Reduction (c): Alternative techniques: Continuous (weight) traction may be used to overcome muscle tension and unlock overriding facets. Control the *direction* of traction with the position of the traction pulley, or by pads under the head or shoulders. The *amount* of traction can be adjusted by the weights: allow 10 lb (4.5 kg) for the head + 5 lb (2.3 kg) for each interspace above: e.g. 35 lb (16 kg) for C5 on C6. The *duration* of maximal traction is monitored by radiographic progress.

53. Reduction (d): A better arrangement is for traction to be applied with the patient in a sitting-up position. Traction is more efficient, being countered by the body weight; the patient can see what is going on, and if paraplegic, breathing is easier as the diaphragm is unobstructed. A framework of slotted angle (e.g. Dexion™) (1) may be attached to the mattress frame if the hospital bed has not this facility, and the frame may be racked up and down (2) while pressure points are being attended to. The weight required (3) should be in the order of that detailed in the previous frame. The line of traction should start in the neutral position or slight flexion (4). The patient should be sedated, *and in the recently injured patient radiographs to check progress should be taken every 15 minutes.* Failure to reduce after several hours is often regarded as an indication for an open procedure.

54. Reduction (e): As soon as the neck has been stretched sufficiently to allow the locked facets just to clear one another (2), the neck should be extended to complete the reduction (3) and traction reduced. In long standing cases (say 1–3 weeks post injury) progress will be much slower, and in extreme cases can extend to days. Generally, if reduction is not achieved after 6 hours, manipulative or open reduction is advised rather than increasing the amount or duration of traction.

55. Reduction (f): The radiograph on the left shows an unstable dislocation of C6 on C7, with locked facets and an associated fracture of the spinous process of C6. On the right the dislocation has been reduced. The C6/7 disc space indicates that further reduction of traction is required. **Aftercare:** If the original injury was confined to the posterior ligament complex, then to avoid late subluxation a posterior segmental cervical fusion is necessary. If the instability is due to a *fracture* (as above) and healing of that fracture will restore stability, then it is sufficient to support the neck until union occurs. This may be achieved by continuous traction (in the order of 2.5 kg (6 lb), taking care that on no account should the neck be over distracted). Alternatively, depending on your assessment of the degree of inherent residual instability and local practice, you may use a halo vest, an extensive off the shelf brace, casts, or internal fixation. Note, however, that at the end of any period of conservative treatment *stability must be checked with flexion and extension laterals.*

56. The halo vest (a): The halo (h) may be attached to a vest (or cast), with additional components. On each side, a transverse bar (tb) is screwed (s) to the halo. These in turn are fixed to 4 uprights (u) with locking couplings (lc). The caudal ends of the uprights are attached through additional couplings fixed to plastic connectors (pc). These may form integral parts of a vest, or be incorporated in a plaster cuirass or jacket.

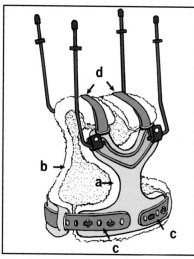

57. The halo vest (b): The Bremer vest has (a) anterior and (b) posterior shells with soft replaceable liners. They are linked inferiorly with thoracic bands (c) secured to locking posts. Above, two shoulder pads which extend from the posterior shell are secured in front with webbing straps (d) which pass through keepers and are fixed superiorly with Velcro fasteners. A range of sizes, including one for paediatric use is available. A pelvic girdle attachment may be fixed to the vest for additional stability.

58. Attaching the vest: The head is supported and lifted up with the trunk so that the posterior section of the vest (with its paired uprights and transverse bars in place), can be slid into position. The transverse bars are then attached to the halo. The anterior shell is now placed on the chest, and the two parts joined together by tightening the thoracic bands and securing the shoulder straps. The transverse bars are attached to the front uprights and the connectors tightened. After check radiographs, alterations in alignment and traction (using the adjusters on the uprights) may be made. Aftercare: 1. Re-tighten the halo pins after 36 hours. Subsequently a loose pin may be tightened if resistance is met – otherwise insert a new pin, tighten it, and remove the old. 2. Clean the areas round the pins daily with soap and water, and remove any crusting with hydrogen peroxide. 3. Treat infected pin tracks with antibiotics and intensified site care. If there is no improvement, introduce a new pin at a fresh site, before removing the old and if necessary carrying out a local debridement. Other complications: These include skin necrosis, osteomyelitis of the skull; extradural haematoma; extradural, subdural and cerebral abscess. Symptoms include headache, pyrexia, fits, hemiplegia and coma. Treat the complication, abandon skull traction, and use an alternative such as a Minerva plaster.

59. Plaster fixation in cervical spine injuries (a): Plaster fixation is occasionally indicated, giving more support than a well-fitting collar. It may be helpful in treating the poorly motivated patient who is tempted to remove a brace. It may also be used in some cases where pin track infections prevent continuation of treatment in a halo vest. Stockingette is applied to the head and trunk (1), and wool padding to pressure areas (2). Felt pads to the chin and occiput are advisable.

60. Plaster fixation (b): Four plaster slabs are prepared from 15 cm (6″) plaster bandages; two are applied over the shoulders (3), one from midscapular region to the occiput (4) and one over the point of the chin on to the chest (5). The slabs are joined with circular bandages; the stockingette and wool are turned down and trimmed (6). This plaster is best applied with the patient seated on a stool.

61. The Minerva plaster: This extensive plaster, although perhaps not giving quite as much support as a well fitting halo vest with a pelvic attachment, is sometimes used as an alternative, especially in children. It may also be used where pin track infections prevent further use of a halo. *Method:* A plaster jacket is applied first (1); this is extended with slabs to form a collar (2); additional support is provided with a head band (3) and side struts (4). If it is to be worn for any length of time, the head should be cropped or shaved (5).

62. (Mid) cervical fusion (a): Under the circumstances of an uncomplicated posterior ligament complex rupture, fusion within a few days of injury is advised. Anterior cervical fusion is somewhat unreliable, and a posterior fusion is to be preferred. *Note:* Traction is maintained during the procedure (1). After carefully controlled intubation, the patient is turned to the prone position, with the head supported in a head ring (2). The cervical spines are exposed through a midline incision (3).

63. Cervical fusion (b): If preliminary traction has failed to obtain a reduction, this may generally be achieved by local trimming of those parts of the facets which are blocking reduction (facetectomy). Failure to obtain reduction is unusual in recent injuries, but there may be difficulty after 3–4 weeks. Note that in very long-standing dislocations, spinal stability is more important than accurate reduction, and the spine may be fused in the dislocated position if reduction cannot readily be obtained.

64. Cervical fusion (c): The ruptured posterior ligament is identified and the adjacent spinous processes, laminae and facet joints rawed. The safest and easiest way to perform fixation techniques is wiring of adjacent spinous processes, either by plain wire (Illus) or Songer cables. Two iliac bone grafts are placed (and sometimes wired together) on either side of the spines, bridging them. Cancellous bone chips are packed into the area before closure. The AO Group favour H-shaped cortical bone grafts.

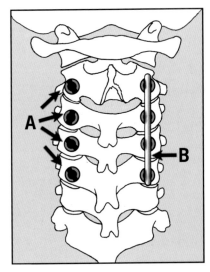

65. Cervical fusion (d): There are a number of other fixation techniques along with bone grafting for cervical spine fusions: Hook plates, similar in concept to Zuelzer plates, may be used, one on each side of the spinous processes. In practice each is bent so that its hook portion can slip under the inferior edge of a lamina, suitably notched to receive it and to prevent it from drifting; its upper end is held with a single screw into the articular mass. A Bosworth H-graft (Illus.) with cancellous bone chips may then be applied.

66. Cervical fusion (e): Songer multifilament cables, of stainless steel or titanium, are easier to handle and less prone to failure than plain wires. They may be passed round adjacent laminae, tensioned, and then held with crimps (i); they may be passed through holes drilled through the spinous process bases and incorporate cortical bone grafts (ii); where fixation of more than two vertebrae is required the repair may be reinforced with rods, moulded to lie snugly and held with sublaminar cables.

67. Cervical fusion (f): The DePuy Summit™ spinal fixation system involves the insertion of Minipolyaxial screws (A), into the lateral masses of the vertebrae (but with the option of pedicle insertion). These screws must be sited with great accuracy, using a clearly established technique that will ensure the vertebral arteries and nerve roots are not compromised. The slots in the head caps are then aligned to take connecting rods (B). These must be cut to an appropriate length and bent so that they bed into the head slots.

1. No posterior mid-line tenderness
2. No intoxication (which may mask the complaints and findings)
3. Normal level of alertness
4. No focal neurological signs
5. No painful, distracting injuries.

This is generally very reliable, but is not infallible: if in doubt, there should be no hesitation in commencing further investigation by obtaining X-rays of the neck.

Radiographs: If these are taken they may show the following: 1. There may be loss of the usual cervical curvature or localised kinking (of greater significance). 2. Occasionally there may be evidence of hyperextension (anterior osteophytic avulsion) or hyperflexion (flake fracture of a spinous process). 3. The presence of pre-existing osteoarthritic changes in the cervical spine which predispose to injury (by concentrating local stresses) should be noted.

MRI scans: These are frequently performed, and may show evidence of disc prolapse or nerve root compression. The results, however, can be unreliable, as abnormalities have been reported in symptomless patients, and vice versa.

Treatment: Treatment is primarily conservative, and to minimise the risks of the superimposition of a non-organic element, a positive approach in the handling of these cases, with emphasis of the likelihood of a complete recovery, is strongly advised. It has been suggested that the content of any medico-legal report in the early stages (and which the patient is likely to see) should reflect this.

The Quebec study strongly advised against the prolonged use of cervical collars, which they considered to be associated with cases with poorer outcomes. They advocate:

Grade I: Immediate return to normal activities, with no work restrictions and no medication.
Grade II: To return to normal activities as soon as possible, and preferably within a week. Temporary alteration of work patterns may be required, but the need for these should be reassessed after 2 weeks unless the clinical circumstances or the working environment are unusual. Non-narcotic analgesics and/or NSAIDs may be prescribed for up to 1 week only.
Grade III: As in Grade II, but narcotic analgesics may be required for short periods initially. Manipulation may be of transient benefit, but not more than two sessions are recommended. Treatment started by a physiotherapist and continued at home by the patient himself is generally very helpful, with emphasis again being placed on the likelihood of a good recovery. McKenzie exercises are considered to be of particular value.

Cases persisting over 3 months: Carefully reassess, and if necessary consider the prescription of minor tranquillisers or antidepressants. Grade III patients with progressive neurological deterioration or persisting radicular arm pain may be considered for surgery provided a disc protrusion at the relevant level has been confirmed: then discectomy and anterior cervical fusion generally give a good result.

Barré-Lieou syndrome: This may follow a whiplash incident. There is complaint of headache, vertigo, tinnitus, ocular problems and facial pain. It is thought that it may be due to a sympathetic nerve disturbance at the C3-4 level, and in 75% of the cases there is impairment of sensation in the C4 dermatome, with weakness of shoulder and scapular movements. Myelography may show nerve root sleeve disturbances. Good results have been claimed for anterior discectomy combined with local cervical fusion.

106. Fractures of the thoracic and lumbar spine:

Mechanism of injury: Fractures of the thoracic and lumbar spine occur most frequently as a result of forces which tend to produce flexion of the spine. A rotational element is often present.

Causes: The many possible causes of this type of injury include:

1. Falls from a height on to the heels, where the direction of the forces acting on the spine are offset by the normal thoracic convexity, leading to anterior stress concentrations
2. Blows across the back and shoulders which cause the spine to jack-knife at the thoracolumbar junction, e.g. injuries in the mining and construction industries
3. Flexion and rotational forces transmitted to the spine from road or vehicle impact in car and motor cycle accidents
4. Heavy lifting, especially in the middle aged and elderly, where there is often the pathological element of osteoporosis or osteomalacia. Less commonly malignancy (especially metastatic deposits) may be a factor, when the causal force may be slight or not even remembered.

107. Diagnosis: Suspect a history of back pain after trauma, particularly if there is local spinal tenderness (1), pain on spinal percussion (2), or especially if there is an angular kyphosis (3). Thoracic or abdominal radicular pain may wrongly divert attention to the chest or abdomen, and in the elderly there may be no convincing history of injury; any suspicion merits radiography.

108. Radiographs (a): AP and lateral radiographs only should be taken in the first instance. In the obviously seriously injured patient there may be difficulty in obtaining a lateral because of severe pain, or through fear of causing cord damage. In these circumstances, a shoot-through lateral may be taken using a fixed grid or chest bucky. (Illus.: shoot-through lateral; note tacks securing canvas to stretcher poles, but detail sufficient to show an anterior wedge compression fracture of L3, with anterior subluxation and obvious instability.)

109. Radiographs (b): If these measures are unsatisfactory you should *personally* supervise the turning of the patient on to his side in order to obtain a lateral projection. In essence you should see that the patient is rotated gently and smoothly in such a way that the upper part of the spine with the shoulders is rotated in step with the pelvis, as in the so-called 'log roll' manoeuvre – with sufficient staff to guide the neck, shoulder girdle, pelvis and legs. You should also see that the patient remains well supported (e.g. by pillows) when he is on his side. This is often a convenient time to physically inspect the back, looking for bruising, swelling and deformity, and palpating to detect tenderness, local oedema and any palpable gap between the spinous processes (signifying a posterior complex injury with implied instability).

110. Note:

1. The most important decision to make in any spinal injury is whether it is stable. This obviously profoundly influences the approach to treatment.

2. *Most stable fractures* are uncomplicated by damage to the cord or cauda equina (although certain *mechanically* stable bursting fractures may be *neurologically* unstable).

3. *Unstable fractures* of the spine may be recognised in the plain films, but if there is any doubt, CT scanning to show the state of the middle and posterior columns and any encroachment in the spinal canal is indicated.

   Unstable fractures may be accompanied by neurological involvement. If this is incomplete, there is always hope of recovery. There is, however, the risk that further displacement at the fracture site may jeopardise this, or convert an uncomplicated injury to a complicated one. Treatment is, therefore, vitally important.

4. The commonest spinal injury *by far* is the flexion compression wedge fracture.

5. In practice, the most frequently encountered problems are recognising such a fracture and deciding whether it is stable or not.

6. Other types of injury are more often unstable than not.

111. Stable flexion compression (wedge) fractures (a): Flexion compression (anterior wedge) fractures are most commonly observed in lateral radiographs and are caused by pure flexion forces. (Illus.: flexion compression fractures of two vertebrae: note the difference in height between the anterior and posterior margins of each vertebral body.)

112. Stable flexion compression fractures (b): Less commonly, when there is a rotational element added to forward flexion, vertebral wedging may be apparent in the AP projection (lateral wedging). (Illus.: lateral wedging of L3 resulting in a traumatic scoliosis.) This form of wedging is often associated with root compression on the narrowed side, and these injuries have a poorer prognosis regarding ultimate functional recovery and freedom from pain.

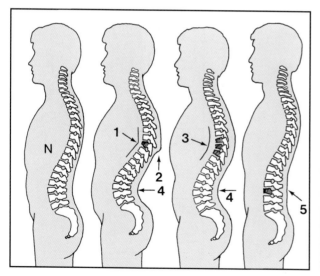

113. Interpreting the radiographs (a): In the thoracic spine, a flexion compression fracture with anterior wedging of a single vertebra will lead to localised kinking (1) with or without a localised overlying kyphotic prominence (2). Multiple fractures in the thoracic spine, especially when wedging is slight in each of the affected vertebrae, will lead to a more regular kyphosis (3). In either of these circumstances, the increased thoracic curvature will tend to produce an increased lumbar lordosis (except where the lumbar spine is arthritic) (4) and/or hyperextension in the hip joints. In the case of the lumbar spine, there may be obliteration or reversal of the normal lumbar lordosis (5). (Compare with the normal profile, N.)

114. Interpreting the radiographs (b): In the commonest flexion compression fractures, the anterior border of the vertebra will measure less than the posterior border. The crushing of the anterior portion may be quite regular, or may result in a marginal shearing fracture (generally the anterior superior corner) (Illus.). If the *posterior* margin appears to show a decrease in height (compared with the heights of the vertebrae above and below) this is evidence of greater violence, and raises the possibility of an element of burst fracture, with the risk of bony fragments encroaching the vertebral canal. If this is suspected, a CT scan to clarify the issue is recommended.

115. Interpreting the radiographs (c): Assess the amount of wedging; the fracture is likely to be stable if the height of the anterior margin still amounts to two-thirds or more of the posterior margin or, putting this another way, if the degree of wedging is 15° or less, or if the width of the body divided by the difference in the heights is greater than 3.75:
(i.e. $x < 15°$, or $c/b-a > 3.75$).

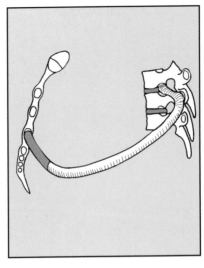

116. Interpreting the radiographs (d): In the case of the upper eight thoracic vertebrae, note any associated fractures of the sternum or ribs. Each of the upper thoracic vertebrae is linked by ribs to the sternum, and *appreciable* wedging cannot take place without involvement of these structures. Involvement of this so-called 'fourth column' is indicative of potential spinal instability.

117. Unstable fractures (a): Marked wedging (20° or more, or collapse of the anterior margin to less than half the posterior) points to damage to the posterior ligament complex, and therefore to instability. (Note, however, that if the *posterior* margin is reduced in height a greater degree of wedging is possible prior to posterior complex rupture – but in the presence of this finding, the possibility of a burst fracture should be investigated, e.g. by CT scanning.)

118. Unstable fractures (b): In this fracture of L1 there is marked anterior wedging (16°) and an associated anterior shearing fracture. The degree of wedging suggests that this is an unstable fracture and likely to be associated with a disruption of the posterior ligament complex. The film has been cut off so that the posterior part of the vertebra and its relationship with the vertebral canal is not defined.

119. Unstable fractures (b) ctd: More information was obtained by CT scanning. This sagittal construction confirms the comminution of the fracture, with an additional clear vertical split through the vertebral body in keeping with a bursting fracture. The height of the posterior part of the vertebra is reduced, with encroachment on the spinal canal. There is no evidence of damage to the posterior ligament complex, so that in spite of initial appearances this fracture is likely to be stable.

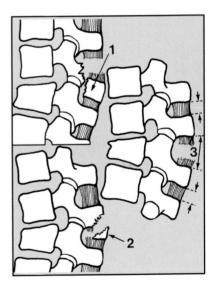

120. Unstable fractures (c): Look for other evidence of damage to the posterior ligament complex and associated structures fundamental to spinal stability. Note especially any avulsion fracture of a spinous process (1), avulsion fracture of the tip of a spinous process (2), and wide separation of the vertebral spines at the level of injury (3). In the cases illustrated, the possibility of the additional involvement of the facet joints should be considered.

The *duration of pressure* applied to any one area is in practice regulated by regular turning of the patient. During the initial weeks of treatment it is essential that the patient does not lie for longer than 2 hours in one position. If the patient is being nursed on a Stryker frame, then he alternates from the prone to the supine; if he is being nursed in bed, then he alternates between lying on each side (being turned a minimum of 40°) and in the supine position. It is important to note that regular turning of the patient should start from the time of injury; irreversible damage may be done on the day of admission when other problems allow this vital aspect of treatment to be overlooked for some hours.

The *amount of pressure* applied to the skin is obviously important: if the body weight is locally concentrated then ischaemia will be complete. If the skin loading is reduced by being spread over a large area, then ischaemia will be less severe and more tolerable. Because of these loading factors, pressure sores tend to commence over bony prominences – the sacrum, the trochanters, the heels, the elbows and the malleoli. Particular attention should be paid to these areas, and local padding over the ankles and elbows may help. To distribute the body weight more evenly, the patient may be nursed on pillows laid across the bed from head to foot. When the patient is lying on his back, additional pillows laid horizontally may be used to support the elbows and arms. Pillows or rolled up towels may also be placed under the ankles so that the heels are relieved of pressure. When the patient is lying on his side, a pillow may be placed between the legs and the legs positioned in such a way that the malleoli and knees are free from pressure. In some centres, water beds, sand beds or ripple mattresses are used to help distribute the loads on the skin, although these on their own are insufficient to prevent heel sores.

It is important to preserve the tone and general condition of the skin. If it becomes moist it becomes susceptible to bacterial invasion. If it is subjected to friction through contact with rough, unyielding surfaces, local abrasions may occur. Local injury of this nature increases tissue demands and may initiate the production of pressure sores. To prevent this: 1. Unstarched, soft bed linen should be used and non-porous surfaces avoided. Nursing the patient on sheepskin is sometimes advocated. 2. The skin should be protected from incontinence. 3. Skin hygiene should be maintained by frequent, thorough cleansing with soap and water. After washing, the skin must be thoroughly dried.

If pressure sores occur, substantial undermining of the skin may conceal the often considerable extent of each lesion. Preventative measures should be tightened up, and any underlying anaemia corrected. Any local sloughs or sequestra should be removed. If the area involved is small, healing may be achieved with local dressings, going through the stages of granulation and contraction. If a large area is involved, rotational flaps usually afford the best means of closure. If sores persist, they are frequently followed by progressive anaemia, deterioration in general health and well-being, and often amyloid disease.

TREATMENT OF THE BLADDER

Note first the neurological control of the bladder detailed on the following frames a–c:

Neurological control of the bladder (a): *Note:* (i) Autonomic fibres controlling the detrusor muscle of the bladder and the internal sphincter travel from cord segments S2, 3 and 4 to the bladder via the cauda equina (1). (ii) Under normal circumstances bladder sensation and voluntary emptying are mediated through pathways stretching between the brain and the sacral centres (2).

Neurological control of the bladder (b): If the cord is transected above S2 (e.g. by a thoracic spine fracture) voluntary control is lost, but the potential for coordinated contraction of the bladder wall, relaxation of the sphincter and complete emptying remains. (Normally 200–400 mL of urine is passed every 2–4 hours, the reflex activity being triggered by rising bladder pressure or skin stimulation.) (Automatic bladder or cord bladder.)

Neurological control of the bladder (c): Injuries which damage the sacral centres (1) or the cauda (2) prevent coordinated reflex control of bladder activity. Bladder emptying is always incomplete and irregular, and occurs only as a result of distension. Its efficiency varies with the patient's state of health, the presence of urinary infection and muscle spasms. (Autonomous or isolated atonic bladder.) In summary, the effects on the bladder are dependent on the level of injury.

Prevention of overdistension The long-term aims of treatment are to minimise the effects of chronic bladder distension such as renal failure, bladder calculi, and chronic infection. The immediate problem is the prevention of overdistension of the bladder while minimising the risks of infection. Indwelling catheterisation is the method of choice, initially with *free drainage*. In the acute situation urethral catheterisation should not be attempted in the presence of priapism, when suprapubic catheterisation should be undertaken.

Mechanical emptying of the bladder by catheterisation is usually required for 3–4 weeks, after which, in the appropriate lesions, automatic function will be starting to take over. A bladder retraining programme may then be initiated. The bladder emptying profile – i.e. when most urine is produced – should be assessed first. A constant fluid intake is adhered to, then the aim should be to provide the most efficient way of emptying the bladder. Ultrasound and urodynamic analysis may be used to judge the completeness of bladder emptying. After an initial IVP, this is repeated at yearly intervals, along with a urine culture, estimation of the serum urea and creatine, and the performance of a creatine clearance test.

TREATMENT OF THE BOWEL

Paralytic ileus is common in neurogenic shock, occurring almost immediately in thoracolumbar injuries but up to 48 hours later in cervical spine injuries. It may be detected by finding evidence of abdominal distension and absent bowel sounds. To lessen the risks of vomiting and aspiration it should be dealt with promptly by stopping fluids by mouth, passing a nasogastric tube, and by intravenous fluid replacement guided by serial electrolyte investigations.

If there is accumulation of intestinal gases then a flatus tube should be passed. To lessen the risks of stress ulceration and gastric haemorrhage, omeprazole or a similar preparation should be given prophylactically.

After a period of neurogenic shock, two types of bowel control problems may be found:

1. In the case of upper motor neurone damage (e.g. T12 and above), reflex activity and sphincter tone are maintained, and the bowel will contract and empty when stimulated.
2. Where the damage is of a lower motor neurone pattern (usually in lesions below L1) the sphincter is flaccid, and faecal retention and overflow of faecal fluid will occur even though peristalsis will return. The care recommended by the British Orthopaedic Association[7] is as follows:

1. Daily insertion of glycerine suppositories 15–20 minutes prior to rectal examination and evacuation if the rectum is full.
2. When bowel sounds return, if flatus is passed, or the bowels move then aperients (Senna tablets and Lactulose on alternate evenings) should be started.

In the upper motor neurone (reflex) bowel, daily rectal examination and manual evacuation should be continued, with suppositories on the mornings after the aperients have been given. Anal stimulation should be employed to trigger the emptying reflex, followed by rectal examination to ensure that this has been complete.

In the lower motor neurone (flaccid) bowel, continue with daily rectal examination and essential manual evacuation.

TREATMENT OF SPASTICITY

With the return of the spinal reflexes spasticity of the trunk and limb muscles may develop. The aim should be to prevent contractures and maintain a full range of joint movements by physiotherapy and appropriate medication: diazepam is often of value.

TREATMENT OF PAIN

Neuropathic pain, often accompanied by disturbing hyperaesthesia may develop at or below the level of injury. This is best managed through the combined efforts of a pain management team.

TREATMENT OF AUTONOMIC DYSREFLEXIA

This condition of reflex sympathetic overactivity may lead to a rapidly rising hypertension which may be severe enough to cause intracranial haemorrhage. It may occur in patients with lesions at or above T6, and be precipitated by a number of factors which include bladder distension (e.g. from a blocked catheter), bowel distension and rectal stimulation (from a variety of causes including rectal examination and fissures), pressure sores and ingrowing toenails, and operations performed without anaesthesia (even in areas which have no sensation). The symptoms at onset include severe pounding headache, profuse sweating, and chest tightness. On examination there is hypertension and bradycardia, dilation of the pupils, and disturbance of the skin circulation above the lesion (e.g. initial pallor followed by flushing or blotchiness). Below the lesion there may be coldness at the periphery, erection of hair, bowel and bladder contractions, and penile erection and emission.

Treatment
1. Elevate the head of the bed.
2. Give 10 mg sublingual nifedipine.
3. Isolate and remove the precipitating cause.
4. Use paracetamol or co-proxamol for analgesia afterwards, *but not aspirin or NSAIDs.*
5. Urgent consultation with a specialist spinal injuries physician: this can be a potentially fatal condition.

OTHER TREATMENTS

Physiotherapy and occupational therapy These measures should be commenced without delay, attention being paid to the following aspects of management:
1. **The chest:** The risks and effects of respiratory infection should be minimised by deep-breathing exercises, the development of the accessory muscles of respiration, assisted coughing, percussion and postural drainage.
2. **The joints:** Mobility should be preserved in the paralysed joints by passive movements. This must be done with caution if there is any spasticity; overstretching must be avoided to minimise the risks of myositis ossificans.
3. **The unparalysed muscles:** These should be developed for compensatory use, e.g. shoulder girdle exercises to make unaided bed–wheelchair transfers possible.
4. **Other measures:** Depending on the level of the lesion the patient may require assistance in some or all of the following areas:
   (i) Regaining balance for sitting or standing
   (ii) Tuition in calliper walking (or gait improvement in partial lesions)
   (iii) Overcoming problems of dressing
   (iv) Help with alterations and adjustments within the home to permit wheelchair use
   (v) Industrial retraining or other measures to help return to employment.

142. Describe the lesion shown. Is the injury stable or unstable?

143. Describe this through-the-mouth view of the first two cervical vertebrae.

144. This lateral radiograph is of an elderly patient complaining of pain in the back after lifting a heavy weight. What do the radiographs show?

145. What does this AP radiograph show? Which two neurological complications are most likely to be associated with the injury?

146. What does this MRI scan show? Is the injury stable?

147. Describe this injury. What treatment would be required?

148. What does this scan show? What complications might you expect?

149. What does this scan show?

ANSWERS TO SELF TEST

142. Dislocation of C5 on C6 with bilateral locked facets. 50% forward shift is present and the injury is unstable. There is no accompanying fracture.

143. There is a congenital deformity of the odontoid process (hypoplasia). No fracture is present and there is no evidence of other injury. The shadow lying above the hypoplastic odontoid process is that of one of the incisors. This is a common finding which is sometimes misinterpreted as a fracture.

144. Flexion compression fractures (anterior wedge fractures) of L1 and L2 and probably L3. Central ballooning of the disc into L4. Gross demineralisation of the spine, probably secondary to osteoporosis or osteomalacia (i.e. these are pathological fractures).

145. There is a burst fracture of L3, with marked wedging, a vertical split through the vertebral body, and separation of the pedicles. The structures most at risk are: (a) the L3 nerve passing through the neural foramen on the wedged side of the spine, (b) the cauda equina within the spinal canal. A CT scan would help clarify how much bony material has been extruded into the canal; in practice, burst fractures in this region have generally a very good prognosis, even in the presence of significant retropulsed fragments.

146. There is a flexion (anterior compression) fracture of C7. There are additional, less obvious fractures of T1, T2 and T3. Those affecting

T1 and T2 are of hairline pattern. There is disruption of the posterior ligament complex, so that the injury is a significantly unstable one.

147. Anterior dislocation of L5 on the sacrum, with bilateral locked facets, and a fracture of the anterior margin of the first piece of the sacrum. This is a fracture dislocation of the flexion distraction type. Open reduction was required.

148. There is an anterior flexion compression fracture of a single thoracic vertebra, with a marked degree of additional lateral compression and lateral displacement of a significant bony fragment. Such injuries are frequently complicated by chronic pain arising from nerve root compression. In this case an additional sagittal construction showed damage to the posterior ligament complex, so this was in fact an unstable injury. Although no significant neurological damage was found, the cord itself was at risk. (The spine was stabilised using pedicle screws with vertical and horizontal connecting rods.)

149. There is anterior subluxation of C6 on C7. The displacement is small, amounting to less than 25% of the depth of a vertebral body. This is in keeping with a unilateral facet dislocation, and this diagnosis was confirmed with additional views.

1. General principles (a): The two wings of the pelvis are joined to the sacrum behind (1) by the very strong sacroiliac ligaments. In front they are united by the symphysis pubis (2). This arrangement forms a cylinder of bone, the pelvic ring (3), which protects the pelvic organs and transfers the body weight from the spine to the limbs. (The dotted line indicates the path of weight transfer.)

2. General principles (b): If the pelvic ring is broken at two levels, the pelvis may be free to open out or displace proximally (1), carrying the limb with it. Isolated (single) injuries of the ring (2) do not have this tendency. This simple concept underlines the main consideration in classifying pelvic fractures, namely to decide whether the injury is *stable or unstable*. Conversely, if there is a major pelvic displacement, the pelvic ring must be broken at two levels even if on first inspection only one is obvious.

3. Anatomical considerations (a): If the pelvis is subjected to splaying forces, the weak symphysis tends to give first (1); with greater violence, the sacrospinous (2), the sacrotuberous (3), and the anterior sacroiliac ligaments (4) rupture, so that the halves of the pelvis can externally rotate. If the pelvis is subjected to vertical shear forces, the interosseous (5) and posterior sacroiliac ligaments (6) are torn, leading to dislocation of the sacroiliac joint and proximal migration of the hemipelvis. In many injuries local fractures replace ligament tears (7).

4. Anatomical considerations (b): The urogenital diaphragm (1) is pierced by the membranous urethra (2), and the bladder (3) lies behind the pubic bones. Fractures of the pelvis, especially in the region of the symphysis and pubic rami, are often associated with damage to the urethra or bladder: rarely there may be involvement of the rectum.

5. Anatomical considerations (c): The pelvis is richly supplied with blood vessels which are frequently damaged by fractures. *Internal haemorrhage is often severe, leading to shock which can be rapidly fatal.* NB: Shock should be *anticipated* in pelvic fractures and merits *first consideration* (see p. 32). In the region of the sacroiliac joint the lumbo-sacral trunk and the sacral nerves are also susceptible to injury.

6. Classification of pelvic fractures: In both the Tile and the AO Classification three clearly defined Types are recognised: *stable* fractures are classified as Type A; fractures which are *rotationally unstable but vertically stable* fall into Type B; and fractures which are both *rotationally and vertically unstable* form Type C. In Tile's widely used classification the subgroups are as follows:

A1: Fractures of the pelvis not involving the pelvic ring
A2: Stable, minimally displaced fractures of the pelvic ring
B1: Antero-posterior compression fractures (open book)
B2: Lateral compression (ipsilateral)
B3: Lateral compression (contralateral)
C1: Unilateral vertically unstable
C2: Bilateral vertically unstable
C3: Associated with acetabular fracture
Diagnosis: Fractures of the pelvis commonly occur in falls from a height and from crushing injuries. *Screening films of the pelvis should be taken* in every case of multiple trauma (especially in the unconscious patient), unexplained shock following trauma, blunt abdominal injury, and femoral shaft fractures. Instability is best assessed by pelvic inlet and outlet films and by CT scan. If the software for 3-D reconstructions (imaging) is available, this greatly facilitates interpretation of the exact relationship of the bony elements involved.

7. Summary of treatment guidelines: There are two clear issues involved in the management of any major pelvic fracture:
1. Initial procedures (IP) to reduce internal haemorrhage. These include the application of a pelvic binder, an external fixator and perhaps a pelvic clamp.
2. Definitive treatment (DT) of the fracture. Both goals may in some cases be achieved by the same measures. The present tendency is for increasing use of open reduction and internal fixation.

A1 and A2: (Tile's Classification):
IP and DT: Conservative treatment may be followed in the majority of cases.

B1:
IP: apply a pelvic binder or external fixator
DT: use an external fixator; or internally fix the symphysis pubis unless there is a contraindication (such as increased risk of infection from a supra-pubic drain).

B2 and B3:
IP: use an external fixator or pelvic binder if the patient is haemodynamically unstable.
DT: displaced fractures, especially where there is pelvic asymmetry (including those with multiple injuries) and patients with considerable pain, making nursing difficult, should be internally fixed. Conservative treatment should be considered for undisplaced fractures.

C1 and C2:
IP: external fixator (and if necessary a pelvic clamp) plus skeletal leg traction.
DT: internal fixation (e.g. by application of reconstruction plates).

8. A1: Fractures not involving the pelvic ring: Avulsion fractures (a): (1): Sudden muscle contraction, especially in athletes, may avulse the anterior superior spine (sartorius) (1), the anterior inferior spine (rectus femoris) (2), the ischial tuberosity (hamstrings) (3), the posterior spine (erector spinae) (4), and the crest (abdominal muscles) (5). The crest and blade (6) may also be fractured by direct violence. In all cases there is localised tenderness, and symptomatic treatment is all that is usually required.

9. A1: Fractures not involving the pelvic ring: Avulsion fractures (b): In the case of the ischial tuberosity, non-union is an appreciable risk, and if this occurs there may be problems with chronic pain and disability. To prevent this, open reduction and internal fixation have been advocated, and this is especially indicated if there is much separation of the fragment (2 cm or more).

10. A2: Minimally displaced, stable fractures of the pelvic ring (a): These like many other pelvic fractures may result from a fall on the side (1), force being transmitted through the trochanter or iliac crest, or from crushing accidents (e.g. from reversing vehicles (2), rock falls, etc.), or through violence transmitted along the femoral shaft (e.g. road accidents, falls from a height, etc.). Other stable injuries may follow anterior compression forces.

11. A2: Minimally displaced, stable fractures of the pelvic ring (b): By far the commonest fracture is one involving the superior pubic ramus. This is seen frequently in the elderly patient following a fall on the side. Osteoporosis or osteomalacia are frequently contributory factors. *This injury is often missed* and should always be suspected if there is difficulty in walking after a fall, and a femoral neck fracture has been excluded. Clinically there will be tenderness over the superior ramus, and pain on side-to-side compression of the pelvis; movements of the hips may be relatively pain-free. Radiographs of the hip may fail to visualise the area and full pelvic films are required. Treatment is by non weight bearing for 2–3 weeks until the pain settles and mobilisation can be commenced.

12. A2: Minimally displaced, stable fractures of the pelvic ring (c): Other fractures of this type include: (1) fractures of two rami on one side; (2) fracture of the ilium running into the sciatic notch; (3) fracture of the ilium or sacrum involving the sacroiliac joint. The nature of these injuries often suggests at least momentary involvement elsewhere in the ring: nevertheless, assuming that they are uncomplicated, they may be treated as in the previous frame.

13. A2: Minimally displaced, stable fracture of the pelvic ring (d): Many quadripartite (butterfly) fractures (1) of the pelvis, and double fractures of the rami with symphyseal involvement (2) are stable. They usually result from AP compression of the pelvis which is insufficient to disrupt the anterior sacroiliac ligaments: the posterior part of the pelvic ring remains intact and rigid, while the loose anterior fragment is only slightly displaced. *Anticipate shock and damage to the urethra*, but otherwise treat with 6 weeks' non weight bearing.

14. B1: Anteroposterior compression, rotationally unstable, vertically stable fractures:(a): These injuries frequently result from run-over incidents where the wheel of a motor vehicle forces the anterior superior iliac spines backwards and outwards (1); they may also occur when the pelvis is compressed by falling rock or masonry which pins the patient to the ground. The ring fails *anteriorly* (e.g. at the symphysis or through two rami) (2), *and posteriorly* (3). The pelvis opens out (hence the term *open-book fractures*).

15. B1 (b): As the pelvis opens out the sacrospinous and sacrotuberous ligaments are torn, and CT scans may show anterior widening of the sacroiliac joints. The posterior sacroiliac ligaments remain intact, so that there is no vertical instability. *Treatment:* (a) Where the posterior damage is minimal and the anterior gap is less than 2.5 cm, treat by bed rest and monitor the symphyseal separation by repeated radiographs. (b) If the separation is greater or there is any significant associated sacroiliac separation, internal fixation is recommended.

16. Internal haemorrhage: Summary of management (see also p. 32): Disruption of blood vessels within the pelvis (most commonly the internal iliac artery and its branches, and the pelvic venous plexus) may lead to substantial blood loss and a falling blood pressure which may be difficult to control. Blood replacement requirements are generally two to three times greater in posterior ring and vertical shear injuries; anterior-posterior and lateral compression injuries are often associated with vascular injury; and in patients aged over 50 years losses tend to be greater.

Any pneumothorax or haemothorax, any external haemorrhage, and any long bone fractures should be dealt with; depending on the circumstances this may necessitate the practice of damage control orthopaedics.

As a first measure in the emergency room, after satisfactory replacement procedures have been put in place, an attempt should be made to stabilise the pelvis and close any gap. This aids tamponade, and reduces the space into which bleeding can occur. Measures include the use of a pelvic binder, the application of an external fixator, a pelvic c-clamp, and femoral pin traction where correction of vertical shear is required.

In some cases these measures along with massive fluid replacements are not enough to prevent haemodynamic instability, and further investigation is indicated to ascertain if there is any intra-peritoneal haemorrhage. This may be carried out by FAST (Focused Assessment with Sonography for Trauma) and/or DPA (Diagnostic Peritoneal Aspiration – deemed positive if more than 10 mL of blood is obtained). Active bleeding, both intraperitoneal and retroperitoneal, may be seen on a CT scan if intravenous contrast is used. The aim is to get the patient to the operating room or angiography suite within 45 minutes, as time influences mortality.

Positive FAST or DPA examinations then indicate that laparotomy should be performed, to deal with pelvic haemorrhage, and to exclude other pathology such as, e.g. ruptured mesenteric vessels and hepatic lacerations. Continued pelvic bleeding should be dealt with by packing and/or embolisation.

Those patients who have a negative FAST or DPA tests and continue to bleed should be considered for arteriography and selective embolisation with steel coils or gel foam. However, in any case where the patient is in extremis a lengthy procedure such as embolisation is inappropriate, and emergency laparotomy and packing are indicated.

In the uncommon case of a severe retroperitoneal haemorrhage, where in spite of a massive transfusion programme losses continue to gain over replacement, exploration may have to be reconsidered. It is seldom that a single bleeding source can be found, the haemorrhage generally arising from massive disruption of the pelvic venous plexus; then, packing of the wound for 48 hours may give control. Occasionally successful results have also been claimed from ligation of one or both internal iliac arteries.

2. DAMAGE TO THE URETHRA AND BLADDER

Incidence Out of every hundred fractures of the pelvis, roughly five are likely to have a urinary tract complication; more than two-thirds involve the urethra. Butterfly fractures are the main cause of urethral damage, whilst displaced fractures of the hemipelvis are generally responsible for the sharp edge of a superior pubic ramus rupturing the bladder.

Types of injury

(a) Rupture of the membranous urethra: Many of the cases are partial ruptures, with an intact portion of the urethral wall still connected to the bladder. Less commonly, with major trauma, there is complete rupture with the bladder losing all continuity with the urethra; this is a distraction form of disruption, with the bladder displacing proximally.

(b) Extraperitoneal rupture of the bladder: This is usually caused by a sharp spike of bone penetrating the anterior or lateral wall.

(c) Intraperitoneal rupture of the bladder: This may result from any pelvic fracture, and is often seen when the bladder is distended at the time of injury.

(d) Rupture of the bulbar urethra: Injuries of this type generally follow a fall astride a bar or similar object.

Diagnosis
1. Suspicion should be particularly aroused if the radiographs show either of the fractures described.
2. The presence of perineal bruising is highly suggestive.
3. The presence of blood at the tip of the penis is diagnostic.
4. If there is no penile blood, and damage to the bladder or urethra thought possible but not probable, the patient should be asked to attempt to pass urine. If clear urine is passed, no further investigation or treatment is required. A positive chemical test for blood in the presence of macroscopically clear urine should in these circumstances be ignored. If after several tries the patient fails to pass urine, the patient should be re-assessed. The palpability of the bladder should be determined and catheterisation considered.
5. Catheterisation carries the risk of converting a partial urethral tear into a complete one, and of introducing infection. A diagnostic catheterisation should be approached with caution: a full aseptic regimen should be followed, and a fine catheter employed. The procedure should be done by an experienced surgeon, preferably the urologist in charge of the management of the patient. Urethral sounds or catheter introducers should not be used. The procedure should be quickly abandoned if the catheter cannot be introduced with ease. If the tap is dry, this suggests intraperitoneal rupture of the bladder; if blood-stained urine is obtained, this suggests an extraperitoneal tear of the bladder or a partial tear of

the urethra; if blood only is obtained, this suggests a major tear of the posterior urethra.

6. If there are strong grounds for suggesting significant damage to the bladder or urethra (e.g. penile blood) a urethrogram should be performed in preference to catheterisation. The end of a syringe containing 20mL of 45% Hypaque is introduced into the urethra and injected; the penis is closed off with the fingers and radiographs taken. If the urethra is seen to be intact, proper definition of the bladder may require 200–300 mL of contrast medium. The following are common findings:

   (a) The bladder shadow is clearly outlined without spillage: *no significant abnormality is likely to be present.*

   (b) The bladder is partly filled and there is extravasation of the radio-opaque dye to the side: this suggests *extraperitoneal rupture of the bladder.*

   (c) The bladder fails to fill, and there is extravasation of the dye into the pelvic floor: there is *rupture of the membranous urethra.*

   (d) The bladder fails to fill, and there is extravasation of dye beneath the pelvic floor: there is *rupture of the bulbar urethra.*

Treatment of injuries to the urethra and bladder

(a) Intraperitoneal rupture of the bladder: The bladder is explored and the tear located and sutured. The bladder is drained subsequently with a Foley catheter.

(b) Extraperitoneal rupture of the bladder: Small bladder lacerations will heal with catheter drainage alone and may be treated conservatively. Large tears are explored and repaired. The bladder is subsequently drained with a Foley catheter.

(c) Incomplete tear of the urethra: If there is evidence of tearing of the membranous urethra, but the bladder is undisplaced, it is possible that urethral tissue remains in continuity. A cystoscopy should be performed and if possible a catheter should be introduced; a suprapubic catheter may or may not be added. Incomplete and complete ruptures can be devastating injuries and should be managed by those experienced in their management.

(d) Complete rupture of the urethra: If the bladder is floating free it must be drawn down to position. This may be achieved by opening the bladder and rail-roading a Foley catheter downwards. After the balloon has been inflated, the catheter may be used for applying gentle traction. The bladder is drained by a suprapubic catheter which is kept in position for several days. The retropubic space may require separate drainage.

(e) Rupture of the penile urethra: An incision is made over the tip of a catheter passed to the level of the obstruction. The catheter is then passed into the bladder through the other end of the urethra. If this cannot be located, the bladder will require opening and the distal end of the urethra identified by instrumentation from above. The urethra is then repaired, using the catheter as a stent. Delayed repairs are in the majority of cases associated with severe strictures (requiring complex urethroplasty), and should be avoided.

3. INJURY TO THE BOWEL

The rectum may be torn in open fractures with perineal involvement, and rarely in closed injuries of the central dislocation of the hip type. Injury to the small bowel (mesenteric tears or shearing injuries of the wall leading to infarction or perforation) may be produced by crushing injuries of the pelvis. Bowel involvement may be suspected in the closed injury by abdominal rigidity, loss of bowel sounds, loss of liver dullness and distension. Exploration and a defunctioning colostomy are essential.

4. RUPTURE OF THE DIAPHRAGM

Routine radiography of the chest should be performed in all major fractures of the pelvis, and the standard AP projection should eliminate this often-missed complication. If a rupture is confirmed, a thoraco-abdominal repair through the bed of the eighth rib should be undertaken as soon as the patient's general condition will permit.

5. PARALYTIC ILEUS

This complication may result from disturbance of the autonomic outflow to the bowel due to the accumulation of a retroperitoneal haematoma. Treatment by nasogastric suction and intravenous fluids usually brings rapid resolution within 2–3 days.

6. LIMB SHORTENING

Shortening of one leg may result from persistent proximal displacement of the hemipelvis (Type C injuries) or from rotation of the hemipelvis in contralateral lateral compression fractures (Type B3 injuries). Clinical measurement of the amount of shortening is difficult: leg length as measured from the anterior superior spine to the medial malleolus is unaffected, heel-blocking techniques are rather unsatisfactory and the measurement of the distance from the umbilicus or xiphisternum to the medial malleolus somewhat inaccurate. The amount of shortening may be judged with greatest accuracy from the radiographs by noting any discrepancy between the level of the iliac crests on the AP film (after making a little allowance for film magnification effects). A correction (raise) should be made to the footwear if there is shortening of over 1.25 cm (½″).

7. NEUROLOGICAL DAMAGE

Neurological damage may involve (a) the lumbosacral trunk at the triangle of Marcille where there are fractures involving displacement of the hemipelvis, (b) isolated sacral nerves in fractures of the sacrum, (c) the sciatic nerve itself as it passes behind the hip. Investigation by CT scan and 3-D reconstructions may be helpful.

Lesions in continuity predominate, and some persistent disability is the rule. Exploration is seldom indicated unless a mechanical cause amenable to treatment can be demonstrated.

8. IMPOTENCE

Impotence occurs in about a sixth of major pelvic fractures, and in about half of those cases in which there is rupture of the urethra. It is frequently permanent. The cause may be due to neurological damage, but some consider this complication to be related to penile vascular insufficiency.

9. OBSTETRICAL DIFFICULTIES

Even in the case of quite marked post-fracture pelvic distortion, natural childbirth is rarely affected to a degree requiring caesarian section. Where there has been a symphyseal disruption, this may recur, persist, and warrant surgery.

10. PERSISTENT SACROILIAC JOINT PAIN

Sacroiliac pain is a common complication of pelvic fractures, especially where there has been clear involvement of a sacroiliac joint (e.g. in open book fractures, Type B1) and may be permanent. Where there has been a sacroiliac joint dislocation, the risks of severe, disabling pain are particularly high and are related to the degree of persisting displacement. In some cases consideration of local fusion is merited.

11. PERSISTENT SYMPHYSEAL INSTABILITY

This is a rare complication and an indication for internal fixation; screening may be of help in confirming the diagnosis.

12. OSTEOARTHRITIS OF THE HIP

Fractures of the acetabulum are not infrequently followed by this complication. It is dealt with along routine lines. Many cases may come to and are suitable for total hip replacement, and prior reduction of a major displacement will render this easier.

13. MYOSITIS OSSIFICANS

Myositis ossificans is seen most frequently after operative intervention or where there is an accompanying head injury. The treatment is along the lines previously indicated.

60. Traumatic dislocation of the hip: The hip may dislocate as a result of force being transmitted up the femoral shaft. This most commonly occurs as a result of dashboard impact in road traffic accidents (1). Note that this mechanism may be responsible for simultaneous fracture of the patella (2) or of the femoral shaft (3). Force transmitted up the limbs from falls on the foot, force applied to the lumbar region (e.g. in roof falls on kneeling miners) and rarely force applied directly to the trochanter may also cause the hip to dislocate. If the leg is flexed at the hip and adducted (4) at the time of impact, the femur dislocates posteriorly (5), internally rotating at the same time (6). In some cases, the posterior lip of the acetabulum is fractured (7). If the hip is widely abducted, anterior dislocation may occur, even without any axial transmission of force (8). The femur externally rotates (9). Note that, if the femur is in some other part of the abduction/adduction range, these mechanisms may be responsible for central dislocation, acetabular floor type fractures of the pelvis (10). A congenital reduction in the normal degree of anteversion of the hip is a common finding in those who suffer posterior dislocations of the hip.

61. Posterior dislocation of the hip – Diagnosis: In a typical posterior dislocation, the hip is held slightly flexed, adducted and internally rotated (1). The leg appears short (2). Few other injuries are associated with the agony accompanying posterior dislocation, and this is almost as diagnostic as the deformity. Pain is less severe if the acetabulum is fractured, and the deformity may be concealed if there is an associated femoral fracture (3).

62. Radiographs (a): The diagnosis is confirmed by radiographs of the hip; the deformity is usually obvious on the AP projection, but dislocation cannot be *excluded* with one view (cf. dislocation of the shoulder); a lateral projection is helpful in confirming the distinction between an anterior and posterior dislocation, and *essential* if no abnormality is obvious on the AP film (Illus.: Obvious posterior dislocation).

63. Radiographs (b): Acetabular rim fractures may be produced by the shearing force of the backward travelling femoral head (see Frame 60, (7)). The fragment may be small (Illus.) when it is seldom of consequence. It may be large or comminuted, in which case there is increased risk of sciatic nerve palsy, instability after reduction and later osteoarthritis.

64. Sciatic nerve involvement: The presence or absence of damage to the sciatic nerve should be sought in every case, and particularly where an acetabular rim fracture is present. Enquire about numbness or burning sensations in the limb and, as a minimal screening, test the power of dorsiflexion in the foot (1) and appreciation of pin-prick sensation in the leg below the knee (2).

65. Reduction (a): Reduction should be carried out as soon as a general anaesthetic can be arranged. The complication rate is lowest in those treated within the first 6 hours of the injury. The key to success is *complete* muscle relaxation; the anaesthetist should be reminded of this and of the need to transfer the patient on a stretcher canvas on to the floor to allow the hip to be manipulated (1). An assistant should kneel at the side of the patient and steady the pelvis (2).

66. Reduction (b): When the patient is fully relaxed (and the administration of suxamethonium chloride (Scoline) just prior to manipulation is often invaluable) the knee (1) and hip (2) are flexed gently to a right angle, at the same time gently correcting the adduction and internal rotation deformities (3). (*Note:* the assistant's hands, vital to the reduction, have been omitted from this and subsequent drawings for clarity.)

67. Reduction (c): The head of the femur should now be lying directly behind the acetabulum and just requires to be lifted forwards. The force required is variable, but great leverage can be obtained by gripping the leg between the knees (1) resting your forearms on your thighs (2) and flexing your knees (3). The assistant keeps the pelvis from lifting by downward pressure (4). Reduction usually occurs with an obvious 'clunk'.

68. Reduction (d): Reduction is often less striking when there is a rim fracture, and when a rim fracture is present (shown by the radiographs) the stability of the reduction should always be checked by downward pressure on the femur. Gross instability is an indication for open reduction and internal fixation of the rim fracture.

69. Reduction (e): Check radiographs should be taken in two planes (and most advocate routine post-manipulation CT scans) to check the reduction and eliminate the presence of loose bodies and any associated bony injury. The following possibilities arise:
1. The dislocation has been fully reduced.
2. The dislocation and a rim fracture have both been reduced, and the hip is stable clinically: *In both 1 and 2 further treatment is conservative.*
3. Although the femoral head is concentric with the acetabulum, the joint space is increased. This should be elucidated further (with a CT scan, tomography or arthroscopy). Persistent displacement of this type may be due to a trapped bone (rim) fragment or infolding of the labrum.
A trapped bone fragment should be removed by surgery, as if left it will lead to rapid onset osteoarthritis. Excision of a trapped labrum is advocated but the grounds for this are less clear; there would seem some justification for a 'wait-and-see' approach.

70. Check radiographs *ctd:*
4. There is persistent displacement of a fracture involving more than 20% of the rim, or the hip is unstable (Illus.: note rim fragment situated near upper lip of the acetabulum).
5. There is a displaced fracture of the rim with a persisting sciatic palsy. Operative reduction and internal (screw) fixation of the fragment are indicated in 4 and 5; in 5, early intervention offers the best chance of recovery. However, it should be noted that the results of rim fixation in children and adolescents are often poor.

71. Aftercare: Some advocate splintage and/or traction to rest the hip in an effort to reduce the risks of complications. A common regimen is fixed (skin) traction in a Thomas splint for 4 weeks and bed mobilisation for a further 2 weeks before weight bearing. (Others, however, advise much shorter periods of recumbency, e.g. of 1 week, and the value of both traction and splintage have been disputed). If there is a rim fracture, weight bearing should be deferred until about 8 weeks' post injury.

72. Alternative methods of reduction: Bigelow's method: Failure to reduce a posterior dislocation of the hip by the method described is uncommon and generally due to insufficient muscle relaxation; nevertheless, if failure occurs, Bigelow's method may be tried. In essence, the hip is reduced by a continuous movement of circumduction which may be broken down into five stages; (1) the hip is fully flexed and then (2) abducted.

73. Bigelow's method *ctd:* After flexing and abducting the hip, the joint is smoothly externally rotated (3) and then gradually extended (4).

74. Bigelow's method *ctd:* As extension of the hip progresses, the external rotated limb is turned into the neutral position (5).
Stimson's method: This is occasionally attempted when a general anaesthetic must be withheld or where there is an associated femoral fracture. The patient is turned into the prone position (1). The end section of the theatre table is removed and the unaffected leg held by an assistant (2). The pelvis is supported by the end of the table (3).

75. Stimson's method *ctd:* The leg is flexed at the knee and held at the ankle in the neutral position (4). The hip may be reduced by direct pressure over the head of the femur (5) or, if the femur is intact, by downward pressure on the upper calf (6). This may be done manually or by the stockinged foot; the latter procedure allows simultaneous application of pressure over the head of the femur as at (5).

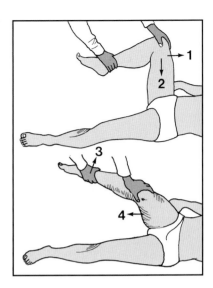

76. Anterior dislocation of the hip: Anterior dislocation of the hip is less common than posterior dislocation. The leg is usually held abducted and in external rotation. There may be swelling and later bruising in the groin. Anterior dislocation may be complicated by femoral vein compression (with the risks of thrombosis and embolism), by femoral nerve paralysis or femoral artery compression. (Persistent absence of the peripheral pulses after reduction is an indication for exploration.)

77. Reduction: Proceed as for posterior dislocation, with the well-anaesthetised patient on the floor, *and an assistant steadying the pelvis.* Flexing the hip (1) and correcting the abduction and external rotation (2) convert an anterior dislocation into a posterior dislocation. At the end of this procedure the head of the femur is lifted up as before into the acetabulum. (The subsequent management is as described in Frame 69.)

78. Reduction: Bigelow's method: This method is less reliable for routine use, but may be tried in the difficult case. Circumduction of the hip is again carried out in the following order of movements: (1) fully flex, (2) adduct the hip, (3) internally rotate, (4) extend, (5) bring into the neutral position.

79. COMPLICATIONS OF DISLOCATION OF THE HIP

1. IRREDUCIBLE DISLOCATION

This may result from in-turning of the labrum or by bony fragments trapped in the acetabulum (Illus. (1)). Open reduction is necessary, *but be certain* that the patient has been *completely* relaxed during the attempts at closed reduction. (Note that if there is a *delay* in excess of 3 hours in attempting the reduction of any hip dislocation, some advocate prior exploration of the femoral vein to remove any thrombus that may have developed, and thereby reduce the risk of embolus.)

2. FRACTURE OF THE FEMORAL HEAD

Osteochondral fractures of the femoral head may remain displaced after reduction of the hip. Small fragments should be excised, but large fragments (Illus. (2)) should be replaced and secured with a cancellous screw or other device. Late osteoarthritis may occur.

3. INTRACAPSULAR FRACTURE OF THE FEMORAL NECK (Illus. (3))

The risks of avascular necrosis are extremely high, and the following treatment should be considered:
1. In the frail elderly, excision of the femoral head, and replacement with a Thomson or similar prosthesis.
2. In the middle-aged, total hip replacement.
3. In the young, open reduction and internal fixation through a posterolateral approach.

4. SLIPPED UPPER FEMORAL EPIPHYSIS COMPLICATING HIP DISLOCATION

Treat as 3 (3).

5. EXTRACAPSULAR FRACTURE OF THE FEMORAL NECK (Illus. (5))

1. The fracture should be dealt with first by open reduction and internal fixation. This can be taxing due to difficulty in interpreting control films in unfamiliar planes of rotation.
2. The dislocation may then be reduced, usually with ease, by closed manipulation; alternatively, open reduction may be considered.

6. FRACTURE OF THE FEMORAL SHAFT (Illus. (9))

1. It is sometimes possible (and especially where there are indications for damage control orthopaedics) to treat both injuries conservatively, reducing the hip dislocation by Stimson's method and treating the femoral fracture in a Thomas splint.
2. If Stimson's method fails, it may be possible to apply sufficient traction to the upper fragment by a substantial threaded screw inserted into the greater trochanter percutaneously.
3. It is generally more satisfactory to expose the femoral shaft and reduce the dislocation by means of a heavy duty bone clamp applied directly to the upper fragment (temporarily insert a large diameter intramedullary nail into the proximal fragment to prevent the bone being crushed with the clamp, and use the linea aspera for orientation). Thereafter the femoral shaft may be internally fixed. (Plating is thought to carry a lesser risk of being complicated by myositis ossificans than intramedullary nailing in this particular situation, although many prefer the latter with cross screwing.)

7. FRACTURE OF THE PATELLA AND OTHER KNEE INJURIES (Illus. (7))

Examination of both knees is mandatory in all hip dislocation cases. Fracture of the patella may be suspected by the presence of bruising at the front of the knee and swelling. Where radiographs confirm that the patella has been fractured, the hip dislocation should be reduced first by any of the methods described and the knee injury treated on its own merits (e.g. a comminuted fracture of the patella should be treated by excision).

Pain in the ipsilateral knee is common (said to be as high as 75%) in patients who have suffered hip dislocations, and MRI imaging has been advocated in all cases. Effusion, bone bruising, and meniscal tears have been found complicating many cases.

8. SCIATIC NERVE PALSY

This complicates about 10% of dislocations of the hip. Fortunately three out of four are incomplete, and about half recover completely.

If no improvement follows reduction of the hip, exploration is advisable within the first 24 hours of injury if there is a large or comminuted rim fracture which may possibly be causing persistent local pressure on the nerve. In other cases the indications for exploration are less clear, and some treat this complication expectantly by conservative methods. (If the patient is being treated in a Thomas splint, this should be fitted with a foot piece to hold the ankle in the neutral position. When the patient is mobilised, a drop foot splint may be required and precautions must be taken to avoid trophic ulceration in the foot.) Others advocate exploration in all cases where a sciatic palsy is still present after reduction, considering that if no other pathology is found, decompression of any haematoma in the region of the nerve will facilitate recovery.

9. AVASCULAR NECROSIS

The inevitable tearing of the hip joint capsule accompanying dislocation of the hip may disturb the blood supply to the femoral head; in about 10% of cases this may lead to avascular necrosis. Dynamic MRI scanning of the hip (using an intravenous paramagnetic contrast agent) gives a good assessment of the blood supply of the femoral head when performed as early as 48 hours after the injury. Radiographic changes however are slow to appear – usually, but not always within 12 months of injury. Clinically, persistent discomfort in the groin and restriction and pain on internal rotation are suggestive of this complication. Avascular necrosis of the head of the femur leads to secondary osteoarthritis of the hip. It is thought that forage arthroplasty (where the femoral head is drilled), if carried out before there is subchondral bone collapse, may encourage re-vascularisation.

10. SECONDARY OSTEOARTHRITIS OF THE HIP

This is the inevitable sequel to avascular necrosis, but may also occur when dislocation of the hip is accompanied by a fracture involving the articular surfaces. (Failure to observe such an injury may be prevented by performing an early CT scan.) It is also seen in cases where scoring of the femoral head is observed in open reductions.

It may occur as a late complication, sometimes as long as 5–10 years after injury; the cause then is less clear, but may possibly be due to articular cartilage damage concurrent with the initial injury. (An MRI scan at an early stage may sometimes confirm potentially harmful articular cartilage damage.) The incidence of secondary osteoarthritis rises to nearly 40% in manual workers who continue with their former occupation. In the young patient, hip fusion may be considered, but generally total hip replacement is the treatment of choice.

11. RECURRENT DISLOCATION

This complication is rare; operative fixation of a large acetabular rim fragment in the hip which is demonstrated to be unstable clinically, may largely avoid it. Otherwise a bone-block type of repair may have to be considered.

12. MYOSITIS OSSIFICANS

This is seen most frequently following exploration of the hip, or when the dislocation is accompanied by head injury. It may lead to virtual fusion of the hip. The risk of this complication ensuing may be minimised in the following ways:
1. Avoid surgery if possible, but if surgery is essential, then the prophylactic use of indomethacin should be considered (see Ch. 5).
2. Splint the hip following reduction.
3. Avoid passive movements of the hip in the head injury case with limb spasticity. Late excision (say after 1 year) of a discrete bone mass, with prophylactic radiotherapy may restore function, but the recurrence rate in other circumstances is high.

13. LATE DIAGNOSED DISLOCATION

This is a euphemism for missed dislocation. Always suspect dislocation of the hip as a possible accompaniment of fracture of the patella or femur.
1. If discovered within a week of injury manipulation may be attempted.
2. After a week and up to several months good results have been claimed by heavy (up to 18kg) skeletal traction for up to 3 weeks under sedation. When radiographs show the femoral head level with or a little beyond the acetabulum, the leg is placed in abduction and the traction decreased; this is generally successful in restoring the head to the acetabulum. If this fails, open reduction may be attempted; in either case pessimism regarding the eventual outcome is often unjustified, many cases achieving a good result without avascular necrosis ensuing.
3. After a year open reduction is unlikely to be feasible and an upper femoral (Schanz) osteotomy may be considered.

80. Slipped upper (proximal) femoral epiphysis: This condition occurs in adolescence; the term is to some extent a misnomer as in fact it is the femoral shaft which moves proximally (1) and externally rotates (2) on the epiphysis. Only occasionally in advanced cases is there movement of the epiphysis relative to the acetabulum (3). There is never any juxta-epiphyseal fracture (i.e. it is a Salter–Harris Type I lesion).

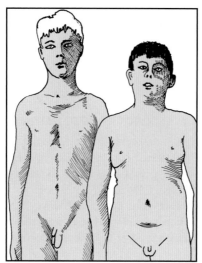

81. Aetiology: Both biochemical and mechanical factors may be involved. *Biochemical/hormonal factors* have long been suspected for the following reasons: 1. The condition is commoner in males, and virtually unknown in females after the menarche; 2. It occurs at adolescence; 3. Those affected are often adipose and sexually immature, showing features of the Frohlich's syndrome, or are very tall and thin, suggesting increased

production of growth hormone; and it is common in children who are receiving growth hormone supplements; 4. Some cases are associated with juvenile hypothyroidism (with lowered thyroxin and thyroid-stimulating hormones), or hypogonadism; 5. It is often bilateral, and 6. In less than 30% is there a history of injury. (There is no hereditary tendency.)

Mechanical factors may include 1. Increased femoral anteversion; 2. Increased obliquity of the epiphyseal plate (physis); 3. Increased acetabular depth; 4. Increased shear stresses on the epiphyseal plate secondary to obesity.

Classification (a): The traditional classification recognises four categories: 1. pre-slip; 2. acute slip; 3. chronic slip; 4. acute on chronic slip.

Pre-slip: there is a history of leg weakness, pain in the groin or knee especially on exertion, and some loss of internal rotation in the hip. Some widening of the epiphyseal plate may be detected in the radiographs, but nothing else.

Acute: the duration of symptoms is less than 3 weeks. There is restriction of movements in the hip, often with an external rotation deformity, and pain may prevent weight bearing. There may be a history of a traumatic incident, but this is often of a trivial nature. The radiographs show evidence of slipping.

Chronic: there is a history of pain in the groin or knee in excess of 3 weeks. (Symptoms have usually been present for months or even years.) There is restriction of movements in the hip in several planes, and in severe cases there may be shortening and an external rotation deformity. Radiographs confirm slipping, and there may be evidence of remodelling and new bone formation.

Acute on chronic: there is a long history of chronic disability on which are superimposed acute symptoms (due to an increase in the slip).

Classification (b): Two more recent classifications (clinical and radiographic) are of prognostic value, and differentiate between so-called stable and unstable slips.

Clinical classification: A stable slip is said to be present when walking (albeit with crutches) is possible. In unstable slips walking, even with crutches, is not possible, and this group has the worst prognosis.

Radiographic classification: Attention is paid to the presence or absence of a hip joint effusion on an ultrasound examination, and to the presence or absence of metaphyseal remodelling in the plain radiographs. In the stable slip, there is no effusion, but evidence of remodelling; in the unstable slip there is an effusion and no remodelling suggesting that there has been an acute event.

82. Diagnosis (a): The condition should be *suspected* in any adolescent with a history of limp and occasional groin or knee pain, especially if overweight or belonging to one of the body types described. Examination of the hip shows loss of internal rotation, often accompanied by pain, at every stage in the condition. In severe cases there is restriction of flexion and abduction; the limb is held in external rotation; and there may be some shortening.

83. Diagnosis (b): The earliest radiographic signs are to be found in the lateral projection. A line drawn up the centre of the neck should normally bisect the epiphyseal base of the head; if it fails to do so, a slip is present, and the percentage and angle of the slip should be noted. (Illus. 15–20%, 17° slip.) **Mild slip:** less than a third, or 30°. **Moderate slip:** 33–50% or 30–50°. **Severe slip:** more than 50% or 50°.

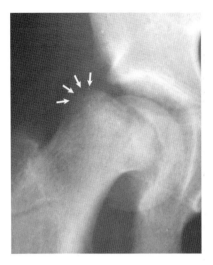

84. Diagnosis (b): In the AP view slip is less obvious, but nevertheless may be detected with experience. Radiographs of both hips should be taken to allow comparison and detect an early silent slip on the other side. In the normal hip (1) a tangent to the neck should cut through a portion of the epiphysis. When slip is present (2) this is no longer the case. (A similar construction (with similar findings) may be used in the lateral, with a line drawn tangent to the posterior part of the neck.)

85. Diagnosis (c): Look for radiographic evidence of new bone formation (buttressing). This may be found in the region of the inferior and posterior aspects of the metaphysis. The latter is shown in the illustration, lying between the dotted line (which denotes the original line of the neck), and the arrows. This finding is indicative of chronicity. A gap between the upper part of the neck and the epiphysis (anterior physeal separation) indicates a high risk of avascular necrosis.

86. Diagnosis (d): Remodelling at the superior (illustrated) and anterior aspects of the metaphysis also indicates chronicity. An ultrasound examination should be carried out; the presence of an effusion indicates a superimposed acute episode. These radiographic features along with the patient's ability to weight bear should allow the slip to be classified as stable or unstable. Finally CT and MRI scans may help diagnose early avascular necrosis and chondrolysis.

87. Treatment (a): The aim is to stabilise the slip and avoid avascular necrosis and chondrolysis. In stable cases, where slips are generally not severe, in situ fixation is advised using a single percutaneous cannulated screw (6.5 to 7.4 mm) inserted through a small incision carefully placed so that the screw lies in the centre of the head perpendicular to the physis, without penetrating the head postero-superiorly (and thereby endangering the capital blood supply or risking chondrolyis).

88. Treatment (b): In unstable cases with severe slipping there is controversy over management. Many advocate pinning in situ; others perform an open reduction or a manipulation. Both are said to be associated with an increased incidence of avascular necrosis and the former is probably best avoided. Any attempts at manipulation must be mild, applying *light* traction in mid abduction and turning the leg into internal rotation. Accept any correction to 30% or less, and pin in that position. *Never attempt to correct a chronic slip.*

89. Treatment (c): Other methods include: (i) conservative treatment, with 12 weeks in a hip spica; this runs the risk of further slipping, chondrolysis, and pressure sores, so it is rarely used. (ii) Immediate corrective osteotomy and internal fixation; the risks of avascular necrosis are high. (iii) *After epiphyseal union, and where there is deformity* a subtrochanteric osteotomy with excision of an anterolateral wedge (1) is a valuable procedure, allowing correction of rotation (2), adduction (3) and extension. This may then be held with a nail or blade plate (4).

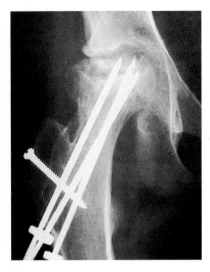

90. Complications: (a) Avascular necrosis: This is a serious complication in the adolescent, and is seen most often in:
1. Acute unstable slips
2. Where there has been over-reduction of the deformity by forcible manipulation, especially where there has been a misguided attempt to reduce the chronic element of an acute on chronic slip
3. Where pins have penetrated the superolateral quadrant, damaging the blood supply to the head (Illus.)

4. Where there has been an osteotomy of the femoral neck.

Treatment: If discovered early (e.g. by CT and MRI scans) a period of non weight bearing with crutches for several months may help to reduce the deformation of the head which occurs through joint transmitted pressure when the bone is soft and in the early stages of revascularisation. Physiotherapy and anti-inflammatories may help optimise the preservation of joint movements.
In the well established case a difficult choice may have to be made between:
1. The uncertain results of osteotomy
2. The difficulty of hip arthrodesis and the risks of late secondary osteoarthritis in the knee, other hip and spine
3. The risks and long-term uncertainties of total hip replacement. (The accompanying illustration is of a case treated by open reduction (with reflection of the greater trochanter) and multiple pin fixation. Neither procedure would be presently advocated by the authors.)

(b) Chondrolysis: This is said to be present if the joint space is reduced on the affected side to half or less of that on the good (or in bilateral cases, a reduction of the space to less than 3 mm). The cause is not known,

but contributory factors include penetration of the head by the fixation materials, severe slips, prolonged pre-slip symptoms and subtrochanteric osteotomy performed prior to epiphyseal closure.

Treatment: This follows the same lines as those employed in cases of established avascular necrosis.

(c) Involvement of other hip: In keeping with the aetiology, the other hip may be affected at any time. This is particularly liable to be missed when the patient is being rested in bed during treatment of the primary complaint. Routine radiography of both hips is advised, particularly in the recumbent patient. If the second hip is involved, treatment is pursued along the lines already described.
Prophylactic fixation: There are some who advocate routine fixation of the other hip, but most consider that the possibility of iatrogenic problems do not justify this unless the risks of the second hip being involved are fairly high. A risk factor of 27% is quoted, but determination of this is a complex statistical matter. Nevertheless this figure is likely to be reached where there is an evident endocrinopathy, renal failure, or risk of inadequate supervision: then prophylactic pinning may be considered.

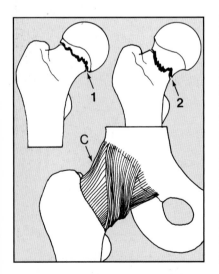

91. Fractures of the femoral neck: Level of fracture (a): Four sites of fracture are well recognised, the most important being: (1) subcapital and (2) transcervical. The distinction between these two is rather blurred, as rotation in the plane of the X-rays may be misleading. It is clear, however, that both lie within the joint capsule (C) and are well described as *intracapsular fractures.*

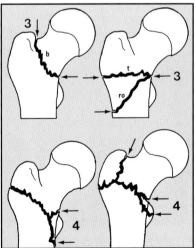

92. Level of fracture (b): The other common sites of fracture are *extracapsular.*
In *intertrochanteric* fractures (3) the fracture line runs between the trochanters. The *basal fracture* (b), the *transverse fracture* (t), and the *reverse oblique* (ro) are varieties of this.
In *pertrochanteric fractures* (4) the fracture line involves the trochanters, one or both of which may be fractured or separated, so that in effect this is often a comminuted fracture.

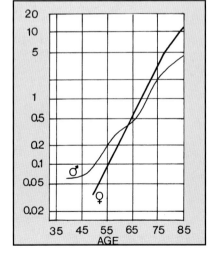

93. Incidence: The *Y*-axis of the graph represents the yearly incidence per 1000 population and shows that below the age of 60 years the fracture occurs most frequently in men, generally from industrial trauma. The incidence increases with age, and in later life is three times commoner in women, where hormone-dependent osteoporosis and a degree of osteomalacia are contributory factors. The fracture is seen from time to time in children.

94. Aetiology: In middle-aged women, a number of factors associated with an increased incidence of hip fracture have been recognised. These include:
1. Having a previous fracture, sustained when above the age of 50 years, following minor trauma
2. Having a maternal history of hip fracture
3. Being a current smoker
4. Having a low body weight.

Mechanism of injury: a fall on the side is the commonest cause.

Risk factors: there are a number of factors (many of which are correctable), which are associated with a higher incidence of this fracture. These include:
1. Poor eyesight
2. Slow gait
3. The taking of hypnotics, sedatives and diuretics
4. Neurological problems including Parkinson's disease and stroke
5. Foot deformities and arthritis
6. Weakness of the lower limbs
7. Loose carpets or slippery flooring
8. A decrease in bone mineral density
9. An elevated rate of bone turnover.

Prevention:
1. The risks of any ageing patient sustaining this fracture should be kept in mind, and any of the risk factors detailed above (e.g. poor eyesight) should be treated as thoroughly as possible. Exercise should be encouraged, and the patient advised against smoking and high alcohol consumption.
2. Calcium and Vitamin D supplements in the elderly, especially if housebound, are cost-effective in reducing the incidence of this fracture.
3. In post-menopausal women, HRT (hormone replacement therapy) should be considered if the patient is known to be suffering from osteoporosis or is otherwise in a high-risk category
4. Where the risks are considered to be particularly high, and low bone mineral density has been discovered, bisphosphonates may be considered.
5. Where the patient is very frail, and particularly if there is any unsteadiness of gait, the wearing of padded under garments (e.g. 'HipSavers') has been demonstrated to dramatically reduce the incidence of these fractures.

95. Diagnosis (a): Inability to bear weight after a fall, particularly in an elderly patient, with or without pain in the hip, is most likely to be due to this common fracture which must be excluded in every case by radiographic examination; fractures of the pubic rami or distal limb fractures are less common causes of this primary complaint. External rotation of the limb, sometimes with a little shortening, is a valuable (but not invariable) sign.

96. Diagnosis (b): *Tenderness* will be found over the femoral neck anteriorly (1) and in extracapsular fractures over the greater trochanter. *Pain* is produced by rotation of the hip (2). *Bruising* (3) is a *late* sign in extracapsular fractures, and is absent in acute injuries and in intracapsular fractures. Rarely, with an undisplaced fracture, the patient may be able to bear weight.

97. Diagnosis (c): An AP radiograph of the pelvis with a lateral of the affected hip are best for screening of this area. Generally the fracture line is obvious but if not, look for asymmetry in Shenton's lines (1) and in the lateral, angulation of the head with respect to the neck (2) or fragmentation (3). If there is any remaining doubt, a localised AP view should be taken; if this appears negative, a T1 weighted MRI image sequence should be obtained to show bone oedema – or a bone scan performed after 48 hours. Otherwise repeat the plain films after 1–2 weeks.

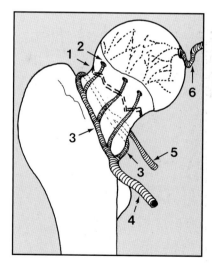

98. Intracapsular fractures: Complications: These fractures are prone to complications for two clear reasons: (a) The blood supply to the femoral head may be disturbed by intracapsular fractures (1), leading to *avascular necrosis*. A dynamic MRI bone scan gives the earliest indication of this complication. Note the main supply penetrates the head close to the cartilage margin (2) and arises from an arterial ring (3) fed from the lateral and medial femoral circumflex arteries (4 and 5). A small portion of the head is inconstantly supplied via the ligamentum teres (6).

99. Complications *ctd*: (b): The head fragment is often a shell containing fragile cancellous bone, and affords poor anchorage for any fixation device. Inadequate fixation may lead to *non-union*. Note that any connection between non-union and avascularity is tenuous – the head is often viable in non-union, and avascular necrosis is seen most frequently in united fractures.

100. Complications *ctd*: It follows that complications are most frequent in proximally situated and displaced fractures. Any displacement should be assessed along the lines laid down by Garden which amongst other things take into account disturbance of the weight-carrying trabeculae radiating from the calcar femorale. *In Garden Type I fractures*, the inferior cortex is not completely broken, but the trabeculae are angulated (abduction fracture).

101. Garden Type 2 fractures: In Type 2 injuries the fracture line is complete; the inferior cortex is clearly broken. The trabecular lines are interrupted but are not angled. In both Type I and Type 2 fractures there is no obvious displacement of the fragments relative to one another. (The absence of displacement is the only reliable prognostic feature of the Garden, AO and other classifications.)

102. Garden Type 3 fractures: Here the fracture line is obviously complete. There is rotation of the femoral head in the acetabulum, i.e. the proximal fragment is abducted and internally rotated. This may be apparent from the disturbance in the trabecular pattern. The fracture is *slightly displaced*. (Garden Type 2 injury is included for comparison.)

103. Garden Type 4 fracture: The fracture here is fully displaced, and the femoral head tends to lie in the neutral position in the acetabulum. (Type 2 injury is included for comparison.) Garden Type 3 and 4 fractures of the femoral neck carry the worst prognosis.

104. Garden classification *ctd*: The radiograph shows a typical subcapital Garden Type 4 fracture. The femoral head is lying in the acetabulum in the neutral position.

105. TREATMENT

IMMEDIATE MANAGEMENT

In the initial assessment the following points should be considered and where appropriate, documented:

1. **Risk of pressure sores:** Where this is high, a large cell, alternating pressure mattress or similar pressure-decreasing bed should be used: otherwise soft surfaces (e.g. fleeces) should be used to protect the sacrum and heels.
2. **Hydration and electrolyte balance:** Set up an intravenous line and initiate an appropriate replacement regimen.
3. **Pain:** This should be controlled to allow regular changes of patient position and reduce immobility – and hence the risks of pressure sores and respiratory complications. *Pain relief should be administered prior to the X-ray examination.*
4. **Core body temperature:** Any reduction should be corrected and the patient kept warm.
5. **Continence:** Catheterisation may be needed if the patient is incontinent.
6. The patient's **mental state, previous mobility** and **overall function,** and the social circumstances should also be noted.
7. **Medication:** It is not uncommon for elderly patients to be taking medication such as aspirin, coumadin (warfarin) or clopidogrel (Plavix), the anti-platelet agent. As their effects may delay surgery for a week (although warfarin can be reversed with vitamin K), prompt attention must be paid to this potential problem.
8. **The X-ray investigation** should be carried out expeditiously, and if possible the patient should be transferred to the ward within an hour of admission.

SURGICAL MANAGEMENT

1. General principles Intracapsular fractures may be treated by:

1. Reduction and internal fixation
2. By primary replacement of the femoral head (hemiarthroplasty)
3. Bipolar arthroplasty
4. Total hip replacement
5. Conservative measures.

In the case of young and middle-aged adults, most centres advocate closed reduction and internal fixation of all grades of intracapsular fracture. (For the management of fractures of the femoral neck *in children* see Frame 137.)

In the fit, older patient, Type 2 fractures are also usually treated by closed reduction and internal fixation. Type 1 fractures are generally treated in the same way in order to avoid the risks of disimpaction, but in a very few centres, are managed conservatively, reserving surgery for those cases where subsequent disimpaction occurs.

In the elderly fit patient, internal fixation is usually extended to include fractures of Types 3, and often Type 4, the view being that if the complications of avascular necrosis or non-union supervene, the patient will be able to tolerate a secondary procedure (usually a total hip replacement). Where the risks of either of these complications are considered in the otherwise fit elderly patient to be particularly high (e.g. in a badly displaced, proximally situated Type 4 fracture) then a primary total hip replacement procedure may be considered, although in fractures of the hip this procedure carries an increased risk (10–20% risk) of dislocation.

Where the patient is less fit, with a life expectancy of perhaps a few but not many years, where there is poor mental alertness, previously reduced mobility from other causes such as arthritis, and/or the risks of complication are also thought to be high, a hemiarthroplasty or bipolar arthroplasty may be considered.

In the case of the hemiarthroplasty, uncemented stems are associated with a higher rate of thigh pain, poorer overall function, and a higher rate of revision. On the other hand, the use of cement may on occasion cause intraoperative hypotension and elevation of pulmonary artery pressure. The risks of these complications must be anticipated, and may be reduced by lavage of the medullary canal and the use of modern cementing techniques.

In the case of unipolar and bipolar arthroplasties, the latter may give a marginally better result in the more active patients within the particular group where hemiarthroplasty is the treatment of choice, especially after the second year. Recently a prosthesis with a press fit modular stem (which gives secure fixation without the systemic effects of cement) has been used. With this the employment of a large modular head gives the possibility (as there is with some other devices) of conversion at later date into a total hip replacement. When the choice of a suitable device in this category is being made, care should be taken to select one which does not permit dissociation of the components should dislocation occur. (Otherwise an open reduction of any dislocation is usually required.) If such a pattern is not available then in the majority of cases unipolar prostheses (e.g. Moore or Thomson) have in consequence a slight overall advantage.

2. Investigations The following investigations may prove invaluable in assessment and are performed routinely in many centres:
1. A chest radiograph and, if there is a productive cough, a sputum film and culture
2. Electrocardiograph
3. A full blood count, with at some stage grouping and cross matching of blood for surgery
4. Estimation of the serum urea and electrolytes
5. Routine charting of fluid input and output.

3. General treatment
1. *Analgesics* appropriate to the patient and the level of pain should be repeated. *Tranquillisers and hypnotics* may also be required but administered with caution. *Preliminary skin traction* (3–4 kg) is practised in some centres, but its ability to relieve initial pain and minimise further displacement of the fracture has not been shown.
2. *Intravenous fluids* should be continued, with consideration given to any concurrent respiratory or cardiovascular problems. (A raised serum urea is clearly associated with a poor prognosis in femoral neck fractures.) Whole blood or packed cells may be required if the patient is markedly anaemic. The type and quantity of replacement are determined by the urinary output, the urea, electrolyte and haemoglobin levels, and the respiratory and cardiac state. Oral fluids are encouraged.

3. *The physiotherapist* may give valuable assistance in the management of the moist chest.
4. *Nursing* of the highest standard is required if, in particular, pressure sores are to be avoided, particularly in the heavy patient who is afraid to move because of pain.
5. *Antibiotics* may be prescribed where there is a heavy purulent spit or frank urinary tract infection; although treatment may be started immediately, bacteriological confirmation must be sought.

While it has been established that the mortality rate for operative treatment of a hip fracture is higher where the procedure is not carried out within the first 24 hours, delay is justified if it can bring the patient into the optimal medical state prior to surgery.

4. Surgical factors For the lowest mortality and morbidity, the following points should be noted:
1. Both the surgeon and anaesthetist should be experienced in this field.
2. Regional (spinal/epidural) is generally better than general anaesthesia.
3. Posterior approaches with the patient in the prone position should generally be avoided.
4. Antibiotic prophylaxis over a minimum period of 24 hours is recommended.
5. Prophylactic measures against thromboembolism should be taken when appropriate.

5. Post-operative care In summary, attention should be given to the following:
1. Monitor and relieve pain.
2. Give oxygen for the first 6 hours following surgery, and as long as hypoxaemia persists (assessed by oximetry).
3. Keep the patient well hydrated and correct any electrolyte imbalance or anaemia.
4. Give postoperative physiotherapy, especially if there is any evidence of constrictive airways disease.
5. Mobilise the patient as early as possible, and preferably within the first 24 hours.
6. Adopt a multidisciplinary approach to the rehabilitation of the patient.

6. Internal fixation devices A large number of systems have been developed for the internal fixation of intracapsular fracture. None meet all criteria that are desirable in this exacting situation: some have advantages under particular conditions and circumstances, and some in others. Most of the design problems relate to the softness of the bone and restricted size of the proximal fragment; it is often difficult to grip it in a manner that will not further imperil its dubious blood supply, while at the same time holding the fragments in close, reliable and continuing proximity, without penetration of the femoral head or extrusion of the device.

The AO dynamic hip screw addresses most of the difficulties encountered in this exacting area, and it and its variations are in widespread use for the treatment of most femoral neck fractures (but see later for alternative methods). It is inserted like the majority of devices by a *closed (or blind) procedure*, i.e. the fracture site is not exposed (although the fracture, its reduction, and the placement of the device are visualised with the use of an image intensifier).

106. The lateral approach for closed nailing procedures: The patient is placed on an orthopaedic table and the feet secured, either with 10 cm calico bandages to the foot platforms (1) or by the use of foot cases (2). If the fracture is displaced it is reduced by applying traction (3) and internal rotation (in the case of most intracapsular fractures) (4). The position is checked in two planes by an image intensifier (5). If there is difficulty in abducting the sound leg to give sufficient access for the intensifier head for the lateral, some improvement may be gained by slightly dropping the injured leg (i.e. by extending the hip) and raising the other. Alternatively the sound leg may be positioned clear of the intensifier head by flexing it at the knee and hip (6); traction in this position is, however, less effective as pelvic tilting is unopposed. Failure to achieve reduction may be regarded as an indication for a replacement procedure. The incision is made in the line of the femur, commencing between the tip of the greater trochanter (7) and the trochanteric ridge (8); its length is dependent on the build of the patient and the size of any plate; small can always be extended. The incision is deepened through the vastus lateralis; this is reflected with a rugine, and the bone exposed using spike retractors (9) which help control any bleeding. The next stage is to insert a carefully positioned guide wire which is used to guide the definitive fixation device. Ideally it should lie either centrally or slightly towards the inferior and posterior parts of the femoral neck, and pass through the centre of the femoral head (10).

107. Insertion of AO dynamic hip screw (a): An angle guide (1) is used to position the guide wire at an angle to the femoral shaft which corresponds with the geometry of the device. The outer bone cortex is drilled and the guide wire (2) is inserted; its position is checked in two planes with the intensifier. A second guide wire (3) may be inserted well out of the way above the first, in order to steady the head and avoid losing the reduction during the insertion of the device.

108. DHS insertion (b): A device (1) which measures the protrusion of the guide wire is used to gauge the length of the screw required (usually 10 mm less than the distance between the shaft and the head margin). The DHS triple reamer (2) is adjusted to the size of the screw, and used to cut a tapping hole for the screw, a hole for the plate sleeve, and a bevel for its shoulder. If the bone of the head is dense, it may be tapped for the screw.

109. DHS insertion (c): The screw (1) is inserted with a guide (3) and its position checked; flats in its stem (2) which permit sliding must be aligned with keyways in the plate sleeve. The guide wire is removed and the plate driven home with an impactor (4). It is screwed to the shaft (5) with AO cortical screws.
A compression screw (6) which threads into the stem of the DHS screw and abuts on a shoulder (7) in the sleeve may be used to draw the fragments together. A screw parallel to the main screw may be used to prevent rotation.

110. Aftercare: After surgery, fluid and electrolytes should be carefully monitored and appropriate pain relief medication should be prescribed. Give oxygen for the first 6 hours, and thereafter for as long as there is pulse oximetry evidence of hypoxaemia. If there is constrictive airways disease then the patient should have pre- and post-operative physiotherapy.

In most cases the patient can be allowed to sit out of bed the day following surgery. Early (i.e. within the first week) weight bearing does not seem to affect the union of intracapsular fractures in a material way, and should therefore be encouraged as soon as the patient's general condition will permit. Once sound wound healing is underway the patient may be allowed home if her mobility and social circumstances will allow. A domiciliary assessment by an occupational therapist is often invaluable in making a decision in this respect.

Out-patient attendances (e.g. at 6 weeks, 3 months and 6 months), with check radiographs, should be arranged until the patient is independent; thereafter, she should be seen at intervals of 6 months to 1 year for a total of 3 years to allow detection of avascular necrosis which may be late in declaring itself. (Note that if a titanium DHS screw is chosen, MRI scans may be used to detect avascular necrosis at an early stage.)

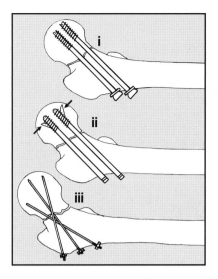

111. Alternative treatments (a): There are many other methods described for fixing these notoriously difficult fractures including:
1. *The use of multiple screws (i).* These have the same complication rate as the DHS device just described, but require a smaller incision as no plate is used. In addition, percutaneous insertion is made possible by the use of

cannulated screws. A minimum of two screws is required. The lower is inserted first, and is positioned so that in the AP view it lies just above the calcar femorale, with its tip in subchondral bone close to the joint line. The second screw is placed as close to the central position in the AP view as possible, and touching the inferior bone of the calcar in the lateral. There is insufficient evidence to say whether there is any advantage to be gained by the use of more than two screws, although this is common practice. If a third screw is being used it should be placed so that it lies as close to the centre line as possible in both the AP and lateral projections.
2. *Hybrid screws (ii).* These have extending wings which are designed to control rotation and backing out from the head.
3. *Moore or Knowles pins (iii).* Three or more are required, and they are particularly recommended in children as their low profile causes the least disturbance to the epiphyseal plate and the blood supply within the bone of the capital epiphysis.
Note that computer-assisted surgery, if available, can be helpful with internal fixation of femoral neck fractures using a minimally invasive technique.

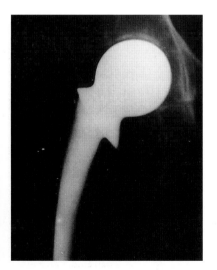

112. Alternative treatments (b): In a frail patient over 65 years, who is not likely to have a long or very active life, and who has a fracture with a high risk of non-union or avascular necrosis (e.g. a Garden III or IV fracture), a hemiarthroplasty may be performed, e.g. with a Moore or Thomson prosthesis (Illus.); the latter is preferred where the calcar femorale is poor. Cemented stems are associated with less hip pain. A Hardinge approach is recommended. There is a tendency to late, slow erosion of the acetabulum.

113. Alternative treatments (c): In the frail elderly patient who has a reasonable expectation of remaining mobile for a number of years, a bipolar hemiarthroplasty may be considered. Where such a procedure is performed the results after 2 years are generally better than those following a uni-polar arthroplasty. The pattern chosen should not allow separation of the components should dislocation occur.

114. Alternative treatments (d): A total hip replacement is appropriate in the fit older patient, particularly with a Garden III or IV fracture, who has medium or high activity levels, or previous joint disease, and has a reasonable life expectancy. It gives better results after 3 years than a hemiarthroplasty, and is the best treatment for a failed nailing. There is a 10–20% risk of dislocation, but if this is an isolated incident a good prognosis can be expected. The most important consideration is the patient's fitness for this more major procedure.

115. Alternative treatments (e): All impacted fractures (Garden 1 and some Garden 2) may be treated conservatively, and this is an important consideration, especially where, in an ageing population, these fractures are on the increase, and where surgical time is in heavy demand. Overall a lower mortality rate has been claimed in those treated conservatively as opposed to surgically.
Method:
1. The leg is rested in a gutter splint until pain settles (usually after about a week).
2. Partial weight bearing with crutches is then commenced, and continued for 8 weeks, after which full unsupported weight bearing may be allowed.
3. Check radiographs are taken 2 days after the start of mobilisation, and thereafter every 2 weeks until the eighth week.
4. If the fracture disimpacts and becomes unstable (a 14% incidence only is claimed) then active treatment becomes necessary, when a hemi- or total arthroplasty may be performed. Disimpaction is seen most often in those over 70 years, especially those in poor general health, or in the younger patient with a low life expectancy. The problems of prolonged recumbency in the elderly may nevertheless follow this line of treatment.

116. Complications (a): Avascular necrosis: In most cases, the cause is the interruption of the blood supply to the femoral head by the fracture. A bulky internal fixation device may further disrupt the blood supply. It is commonest in Grade III and IV fractures. The onset of pain, limp, deteriorating function and restriction of movements may be delayed for many months. X-ray changes usually appear within the first year, but may be delayed for as long as 3 years. The whole femoral head may be involved with increased density, loss of sphericity, joint space narrowing and secondary OA lipping. Changes may show only in the weight-bearing portion of the head ('superior segmental necrosis') where there is a characteristic double break in the contour of the femoral head. Dynamic MRI scans may permit an early diagnosis.
Treatment: Control mild symptoms with analgesics. In severe cases in the young patient a MacMurray osteotomy should be considered; in the older patient a total hip replacement is usually advised. An overall incidence of 15% has been quoted for this complication.

117. Complications (b): Non-union: This is most often seen in Grade III and IV fractures, especially if missed or where the quality of fixation has been poor. In the younger patient, even where the diagnosis is late (e.g. at 6 months) internal fixation and bone grafting (e.g. with a Dynamic Hip screw and fibular graft) may be considered, and in some quarters *primary* treatment with pinning and grafting is recommended for high-risk fractures. The overall incidence is about 5–10%.

118. Non-union *ctd:* In the older patient, especially the untreated fracture where the fracture has come seriously adrift (Illus.), or where there is pronounced rounding of the bone ends, sclerosis, or marked cystic changes in the neck, prosthetic replacement of the femoral head (hemi-arthroplasty), or total hip replacement are the treatments of choice. A Pauwel's osteotomy is a useful procedure both in the young and in the old (up to the age of 70 years) for whom a total hip replacement is a fall-back procedure.

119. Extracapsular fractures. Due perhaps to the decline in the teaching of Latin and precision in the use of language there is unfortunately widespread confusion amongst many surgeons over the terminology of these fractures, and this has now invaded the literature. Reluctantly it must be accepted that it is now probably safest to use the term 'trochanteric' for all intertrochanteric and pertrochanteric fractures, and this has been adapted here. The illustration shows the commonest patterns, graded in order of stability.

FEMUR, *Proximal Segment* : 31–

139. AO Classification of fractures of the femur, proximal segment (31–):

Type A fractures involve the trochanteric area (bounded by the intertrochanteric line and the line separating the diaphysis from the proximal segment, at the level of the distal limit of the lesser trochanter).

A1 = Simple fractures beginning anywhere in the region of the greater trochanter, and ending above or below the lesser trochanter: .1 the fracture runs along the intertrochanteric line; .2 it passes through the greater trochanter; .3 it passes below the lesser trochanter.

A2 = Multifragmentary fractures starting anywhere on the greater trochanter and running into the medial cortex which is broken at two levels: .1 with one intermediate fragment; .2 with several intermediate fragments; .3 with the medial border of the fracture extending more than 1 cm below the lesser trochanter.

A3 = The fracture line extends from below the greater trochanter to above the lesser trochanter: .1 simple oblique; .2 simple transverse; .3 multifragmentary.

[*Note*: Avulsion fractures of the greater and lesser trochanters cannot be classified with other Type A fractures, and have a separate classification, namely 31-D1.]

Type B fractures involve the femoral neck.

B1 = Minimally displaced subcapital fractures: .1 impacted with 15° or more valgus; .2 impacted with less than 15° of valgus; .3 non-impacted fractures.

B2 = Transcervical fractures: .1 basal; .2 adduction pattern; .3 shear pattern.

B3 = Displaced subcapital fractures: .1 moderate varus displacement with external rotation; .2 moderate displacement with shortening and external rotation; .3 marked displacement.

Type C fractures involve the femoral head; they are rare, and are generally seen as a complication of posterior dislocation of the hip.

C1 = Split fractures: .1 avulsion of the ligamentum teres; .2 with detachment of the ligamentum teres; .3 with a large fragment.

C2 = Depressed fracture of the head: .1 posterior superior; .2 anterior superior; .3 depression with a split fracture.

C3 = Fracture of the head and the neck: .1 split fracture with a transcervical fracture; .2 split fracture with a sub-capital fracture; .3 depressed fracture with a fracture of the neck.

Note: 1. The distinction between fractures in Type B is somewhat arbitrary as the great majority of fractures within this group are of a common pattern, the apparent radiological differences being due to differences in positioning or projection.

2. The AO Group observe the following approximate equivalents with the Garden Classification:

Garden 1 = 31-B1.2
Garden 2 = 31-B1.3
Garden 3 = 31-B3.1
Garden 4 = 31-B3.2 or 31-B3.3

SELF-TEST

140. Following a head injury and a dislocation of the hip which was reduced by manipulation, this patient complained of persistent pain and stiffness in the hip. What is the cause of this?

141. Nine months after internal fixation of a femoral neck fracture by a trifin nail this patient complained of pain in his hip.
a. What is the source of his complaint?
b. What was the level of the fracture?
c. Has it united?
d. What deformity of the femoral neck existed before the injury?

142. This radiograph is of a young man who was complaining of severe pain in the hip and difficulty in weight bearing after a sudden sprint while playing football. What abnormality is present?

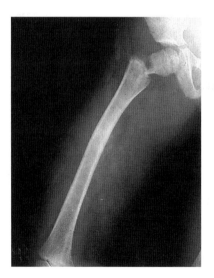

143. This radiograph is of a child who complained of pain in the hip and inability to weight bear after a fall from a tree. What injury is present, and what complications might ensue from this?

144. What does this radiograph show? How would you treat this?

145. What pathology is present, and how has it been dealt with?

146. What fracture has occurred here? What treatment has been carried out? What is the result?

147. What complication is present in this untreated intracapsular fracture of the femoral neck?

148. What injuries are present? How might this be treated?

149. What is this fracture? What complication may be present?

150. What injury is present?

151. What abnormality is present? Assuming this is the only injury, how would you treat it?

152. What class of pelvic fracture is showing in this radiograph?

153. Describe this injury in a child of 6 years. How might it be treated?

154. What class of pelvic fracture is showing in this radiograph?

ANSWERS TO SELF-TEST

140. Myositis ossificans.

141. a. Avascular necrosis with bone collapse.
b. Subcapital.
c. Yes.
d. Coxa valga (secondary to poliomyelitis).

142. Avulsion fracture of the anterior inferior iliac spine (rectus femoris).

143. Delbet Type III (cervicotrochanteric or basal) fracture of the femoral neck with displacement. Possible complications include avascular necrosis, delayed or non-union, and coxa vara.

144. There is a multilocular cyst involving the femoral neck and proximal femoral shaft, with a fracture running across it. This is an undisplaced (as yet) extracapsular fracture of the femur in a case of fibrous dysplasia. The diagnosis would have to be confirmed by biopsy; normally the area would be curetted, packed with bone chips, and the fracture secured with a Gamma™ 3 nail or a Dynamic Hip screw and long plate.

145. Slipped proximal femoral epiphysis. There is some persisting deformity. The position has been accepted (a lateral would be required to confirm the extent of the slip) and held with three pins, one of which may be penetrating the head. Screw fixation might have been a preferable procedure.

146. This is an unstable pertrochanteric fracture which has been treated with a one-piece nail-plate device. This has broken (due to the severe stresses it has been subjected to), but the fracture has gone on to unite, albeit in coxa vara.

147. Non-union.

148. There is an obvious dislocation of the hip. In addition there is a fracture of the floor of the acetabulum. Further radiographs and a CT scan would be required to clarify the extent of the latter, but the impression is of a comparatively undisplaced transverse fracture through the acetabular floor. Assuming this impression is confirmed, the dislocation would be reduced by manipulation; the acetabular fracture would then be reassessed by a postoperative CT scan; if displacement of the fracture is minimal, then conservative management with traction and early hip movements would be advocated: otherwise internal fixation would be advised.

149. This is a quadripartite (butterfly) fracture of the pubic rami; there is risk of damage to the urethra or bladder.

150. This shows a posterior dislocation of the hip which was unstable due to an associated fracture of the acetabular rim; the fragment in question can be seen lying in proximity to the upper and outer quadrant of the femoral head. The hip was reduced, and to maintain the reduction, the rim fragment had to be exposed through a posterior approach and screwed back into position.

151. There is a symphyseal separation of just under 2.5 cm. This should be treated by bed rest until the pain settles. The separation should be monitored by repeated radiographs, and more active treatment pursued (e.g. with the use of an external fixator or by internal fixation) should deterioration occur.

152. Examination of the symphysis shows a degree of overlap. The sacroiliac joints appear intact, but there is a fracture involving the blade of the pelvis and the floor of the acetabulum on the right; the hemipelvis is displaced proximally. This is a Tile Type C3 injury.

153. There is an undisplaced crack fracture of the femoral neck in a child (Delbet type II injury). This might be treated by the application of a hip spica.

154. The right hemipelvis is vertically and rotationally unstable, but the acetabulum is intact: this is therefore a Tile Type C1 fracture. After successful resuscitation the injury was treated by open reduction and held with long cancellous screws and reconstruction plates.

1. Classification: In the AO Classification system the femoral shaft is defined as in effect stretching between the inferior margin of the lesser trochanter (proximal segment) (1) and the upper border (2) of a square containing the distal end of the femur (the distal segment). For descriptive purposes the shaft (or diaphyseal segment) may in turn be divided into proximal (3), middle (4), and distal thirds (5). The proximal third is sometimes referred to as the subtrochanteric zone.

2. Causes of fracture: Considerable violence is usually required to fracture the femur – e.g. in road traffic accidents, falls from a height, and crushing injuries. Pathological fractures may occur in osteoporosis, at metastatic deposits, and in association with hip prostheses. The diagnosis is usually obvious clinically and confirmed with plain films (Illus.). *It is most important to exclude fracture of the patella, dislocation of the hip, fracture of the neck of the femur, and acetabular fracture.*

3. Fluid loss: In a simple fracture, loss of half to one litre of blood into the tissues with accompanying shock is common. Fractures open from within out occur classically in the proximal third. Blood replacement is often required in closed fractures, and normally essential in open ones; grouping, cross-matching and setting up of an intravenous line should be done routinely (except in children). In the transport of patients to hospital, temporary splintage will help reduce local bleeding and shock.

4. Treatment of fractures of the femoral shaft: In the adult, internal fixation by intramedullary nailing is the commonest method of treatment. The prime advantage this has to offer is that it generally permits early mobilisation of the patient, thereby lessening the risks of pulmonary, circulatory, renal, joint and other complications, while promoting muscle activity, joint movements and functional recovery. It may also alleviate problems of bed occupancy (which is the historic reason for its introduction). *Note, however, that nailing may have to be delayed in favour of damage control orthopaedics.* (See p. 44.)

Intramedullary nailing is generally performed using an image intensifier to achieve a manipulative reduction; the fracture is not usually exposed unless this fails. There are many patterns of I-M nail, and much ongoing development. In most cases the maximum possible diameter of nail is chosen after any tight spots have been removed by reaming of the medullary canal. Nails are available for insertion from above (orthograde) through the tip of the trochanter or the piriform fossa, or from below (retrograde) via the knee joint. To prevent rotational instability, most nails allow the use of cross screws inserted above and below the level of the fracture, reducing the need for extensive reaming of the canal and reliance on a tight grip of the nail throughout its length to control this. The original plain intramedullary nail (Küntscher, clover-leaf and other patterns) is now seldom used.

5. I-M nailing techniques (a): Positioning: Careful positioning is required to give proximal access and to allow two-plane visualisation of the fracture with an image intensifier: **(a)** Traction may be applied through foot pieces or a traction pin, on an orthopaedic table with a perineal post. The affected leg is adducted, while the good leg is flexed and abducted at the hip.
(b) Alternatively the operation is performed on a radiolucent table, with a pillow under the buttock (and with or without a perineal post). The leg is positioned by an assistant.

6. I-M nailing (b): Positioning *ctd:* Again, an orthopaedic table may be used with the patient in the lateral position. A horizontal perineal post is employed and used to permit effective skeletal or foot support traction. The good leg is extended at the hip while the affected leg is flexed at the hip to allow access for the C-arm and the head of the image intensifier.

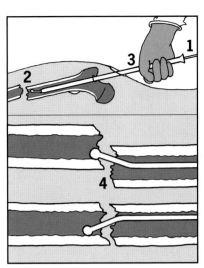

7. I-M nailing (c): Positioning *ctd:* Alternatively, using an orthopaedic table, the good leg may be flexed at the hip and externally rotated, to give access for the image intensifier. Traction may be applied on the affected side in the line of the limb through a Steinman pin (1) through the tibial tuberosity (some prefer the femoral condyles), with the perineal post offering counter-traction (2). The affected side is adducted at the hip.

8. I-M nailing (d): The trochanter is exposed through a 6–8 cm lateral incision; the piriform fossa (1) is identified with a finger, and the medullary canal entered using an awl (2). The position is confirmed with the intensifier before enlarging the opening. Alternatively a guide wire (3) held in the chuck of an introducer may be used and the opening may be enlarged with a cannulated cutter (4). (An easier entry point at the tip of the trochanter may be used with angled nails – see p. 313.)

9. I-M nailing (e): Initially the aim is to reduce the fracture and pass a guide wire (1) across the fracture (2) into the distal segment. To gain purchase on the proximal fragment, a small diameter nail (3) may be slipped over the guide wire. If one angled at its tip is used, this may if rotated facilitate the reduction (4).

10. I-M nailing (f): Reaming is frequently, but not always undertaken before insertion of the nail. This may be merely to remove any tight spots, or it may aim to remove sufficient bone to ensure that ultimately there will be good contact between the nail and bone over a reasonable length of the shaft. Techniques vary, but often a reaming rod is substituted for the guide wire; cannulated flexible reamers of increasing diameter are then fed over the reaming rod until the desired bore has been achieved.

11. I-M nailing (g): The nail is then inserted. (The choice of nail length and diameter is preferably made with X-ray studies prior to surgery.) Instrumentation varies with the devices employed, but generally an insertion handle (1) is attached to the chosen nail (2) and the nail threaded down the guide wire (3). A so-called slap hammer (4) is then usually employed to drive the nail home.

12. I-M nailing (h): Interlocking screws may then be inserted (1,6), but first confirm the absence of any rotational deformity (the second toe, patella and anterior superior iliac spine should be in alignment). The insertion handle usually doubles up as a jig (2) to allow easy placement of the screws. The corresponding holes in the nail may be circular (3) or slotted (4) giving static or dynamic locking (where some telescoping is possible (5)). Distal locking screws may be inserted using the intensifier for location purposes.

13. Retrograde I-M nailing (a): This can be of value in obese patients, in cases of multiple injury, and where there are additional fractures round the femoral or tibial condyles which have to be dealt with at the same time. The knee is flexed over a pillow to about 45°. The intercondylar notch is exposed either through a patellar tendon splitting incision or through a medial parapatellar incision, with lateral displacement of the patella.

14. Retrograde I-M nailing (b): A guide wire is then inserted and its position checked in two planes with the image intensifier. A reamer is threaded over the guide wire, and this is used to prepare the bone to accept the intramedullary nail which may be expanded over a short length at its hilt.

15. Retrograde I-M nailing (c): After the nail has been introduced static or dynamic locking screws may be inserted at the distal end; proximal static locking may also be carried out. Short nails are available for supracondylar fractures (including after some knee replacements) and for some distal femoral fractures after hip replacements. (Illus.: femoral mid-shaft fracture with cerclage wiring and an I-M nail with interlocking screws, plus fractures of the proximal tibia treated by open reduction and interlocking screwing.)

16. Retrograde I-M nailing (d): In the case of ipsilateral fracture of the tibial shaft it may be possible to treat both injuries by intramedullary nailing. In the case illustrated there has been a transverse fracture of the femur in the distal third treated by retrograde nailing and interlocking screwing. In the same session a fracture of the tibial shaft (anatomically reduced and not showing clearly on the film) has been secured with an angled tibial nail, with locking interlocking screws. A vacuum dressing was used to treat a thigh compartment syndrome (note circular ring of staples).

17. Retrograde I-M nailing from the fracture site: Plain, clover-leaf and some other pattern intramedullary nails may be inserted by a retrograde technique after exposure of the fracture. This can be of value where image intensification is not available. The fracture is exposed (1) and the selected nail driven up the proximal fragment (2) until it presents at the buttock where it is delivered through a small incision (3). The fracture is reduced (4), and the nail driven back down (5) across the fracture site into the distal fragment.

18. I-M nailing in children: While conservative treatment is generally advocated for shaft fractures in children, stable fractures of the femur may be treated with Nancy nails (mobilising in 7–10 days) using the principle of 3-point fixation. They range from 2–4 mm in diameter and are flexible. They are bent to fit, and have flattened ends to engage in cancellous bone and control rotation; the other, protruding ends are atraumatic. They are inserted through small 2 cm incisions (medial and lateral supracondylar for mid-shaft fractures), lateral for distal shaft fractures.

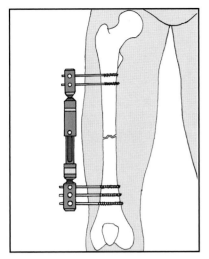

19. Other methods of fixation: External fixators: Fractures of the femur are less easy to control with external fixators than those of the tibia, owing to the magnitude of the stresses at the fracture site from the weight of the limb. Nevertheless the technique is often useful in the management of highly contaminated open fractures, and can be replaced under suitable circumstances by an I-M nail at up to 10 days post trauma. Some cases of open fracture are suitable for treatment by thin wire methods (e.g. Ilizarov p. 79).

20. Other methods of fixation: Plating: This is useful for rapid, rigid fixation in an ischaemic limb requiring vascular repair. Plating has a slightly increased risk of infection and non-union. Compression plating (but see p. 77 for alternatives) is best carried out engaging 8 cortices above and 8 below the fracture, and if possible an interfragmentary screw should be inserted. Compression plating with bone grafting is sometimes used in the treatment of non-union after intramedullary nailing.

21. Aftercare following I-M nailing: Postoperatively, and preferably when the patient is still on the table, the knee should be checked for instability. On return to the ward the limb should be supported on a Braun frame, gutter splint, or Thomas splint. Postoperative radiographs should include good quality views of the proximal and distal femur to exclude any condylar or missed subcapital fractures.

After the first few days care is dependent on the quality of fixation. If a tight-fitting, large-diameter nail is used, and if rotation is well controlled by interdigitating fragments or cross-screws, no external splintage is necessary. The knee may be mobilised and the patient allowed up on crutches. To avoid the risks of the nail bending or undergoing fatigue fracture many prefer to defer weight bearing for 8–10 weeks or until some callus appears. (Shorter periods may be considered when stronger titanium nails are used.) Where the fixation is less sound, a period of a few weeks with the leg cradled in a Thomas splint may be thought desirable.

After union of the fracture, but not before 12–18 months, some advocate removal of the nail in all but the very frail to reduce the risk of a comparatively minor injury causing a fracture of the femoral neck (from local stress concentrations at the end of the nail). This, however, is no longer routine.

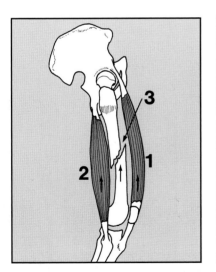

22. Conservative treatment: Femoral shaft fractures may also be treated conservatively, especially in children. If this method is being employed, the first principle to appreciate is that the large muscle masses of the quadriceps (1) and hamstrings (2) tend to produce displacement and shortening (3). Traction can overcome this, and is the basis of most conservative methods of treatment.

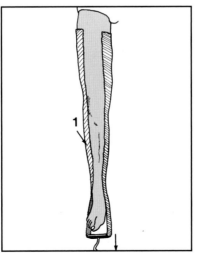

23. Traction methods: (a) Skin traction: Adhesive strapping is used in children and young adults. There are occasional difficulties with skin sensitivity and pustular infections under the strapping, and if this becomes a problem alternative methods may have to be used, e.g. skeletal traction after the infection subsides. (Non-adhesive tapes may sometimes be used for short periods of light traction.)

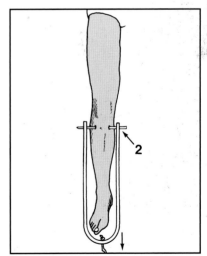

24. Traction methods: (b) Skeletal traction: The site generally chosen is in the region of the tibial tuberosity. (Some, however, prefer the femoral condyles to avoid stressing the ligaments of the knee, albeit this being seldom a problem.) Skeletal traction is preferred in the older patient with inelastic skin and where heavy traction is required. There are occasional problems with pin track infections.

25. Applying skin traction (a): With the exercise of care and gentleness this can usually be done without an anaesthetic. (1) Begin by shaving the skin. (2) It is then traditional to swab or spray the skin with a mildly antiseptic solution of balsam of Peru in alcohol. This may facilitate the adhesion of the strapping.

26. Applying skin traction (b): Commercial traction sets use adhesive tapes which can stretch from side to side but not longitudinally. They come supplied with traction cords (1) and a spreader bar (2) with foam protection for the malleoli (3). Begin by applying the tape to the medial side of leg – do this by peeling off the protective backing with one hand (4) while pressing the tape down and advancing the other (5).

27. Applying skin traction (c): The leg is internally rotated and the tape applied to the outside of the leg, preferably a little more posterior than on the medial side. The tapes should extend up the leg as far as possible, irrespective of the site of the fracture. Now apply traction to the leg (6) and finally secure the tapes throughout their length with encircling crepe bandages (7).

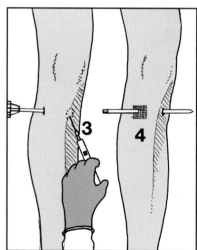

28. Applying skeletal traction (a): The preferred site is the upper tibia a little under 2 cm (1″) posterior to the prominence of the tibial tuberosity (1). It is important to avoid the knee joint, and the growth plate in children so begin by carefully identifying it by flexing the knee (2), noting its relationship to the tuberosity (3). If a general anaesthetic is not employed, infiltrate the skin and tissue down to periosteum with local anaesthetic (e.g. 2–3 mL of 1% lidocaine) (4).

29. Skeletal traction (b): Now make a small incision in the skin (1) enough to take the traction pin only; inset it until the point strikes bone. Drive the pin through the lateral tibial cortex by applying firm pressure and twisting the chuck handle (2). You should feel it penetrate the outer cortex and pass quickly with little resistance till it meets the medial cortex. Stop at this stage.

30. Skeletal traction (c): Infiltrate the skin down to periosteum on the medial side, using the lie of the pin to guide you to the expected exit area (3). Drive the pin through the medial cortex, and make a small incision over the tenting skin to allow it to come through. Protect the openings with gauze strips soaked in Nobecutane™ or a similar sealant (4). Try to inset the pin at right angles to the leg.

31. Traction systems: Skin traction in a Thomas splint (a): The most important decision in selecting a Thomas splint is the ring size. To save time (e.g. before anaesthesia) the uninjured leg may be measured, and an allowance of 5 cm made for swelling, present and anticipated. It is nevertheless wise to have readily available a size above and below the estimate in case of inaccuracies.

32. Thomas splint (b): Anaesthesia will be required in the adult. Applying traction with one hand on the spreader bar (2) the selected splint is pushed up the leg (3). It should reach the ischial tuberosity (or more likely the perineum) and it should be possible to pass one finger beneath the ring round its complete circumference. If the ring is too large or too small, maintain traction while the next size is tried.

33. Thomas splint (c): The choice of soft furnishings and their method of application is often made with a fanaticism that may amaze the uncommitted. Slings to bridge the side irons may be formed from strips of 15 cm (6″) wide calico bandage (1). It is traditional to secure these with large safety pins inserted from below, close to the outer iron (2). Sometimes spring clips are used. A double bandage thickness ensures greater rigidity (3).

34. Thomas splint (d): The sling placed directly beneath the fracture (5) should preferably be unyielding, and one of canvas with web and buckle fastenings (4) is often favoured in this situation. It is customary to apply the splint with the master sling in position; the other slings are then attached and adjusted to the contours of the limb. Less satisfactorily perhaps the splint is applied with all the slings already in position.

35. Thomas splint (e): Calico and canvas slings can drift, separate, or ruck, and many prefer the smoothness of an unbroken circular bandage, stretched in double thickness over the splint (e.g. Tubigrip™) (1). This has the disadvantage of 'waisting' the splint (2), being less than firm under the fracture and tending to drift distally (3). The last may be prevented by anchoring it to the ring with ribbon gauze or bandage (4).

36. Thomas splint (f): If multiple slings are used, any tendency for them to separate may be minimised by pinning each to its neighbour (1); any tendency to distal drift may be prevented by attaching the top sling to the posterior half of the ring. A layer of wool should be placed between the slings and the limb to smooth out any unevenness (2) (not necessary with circular woven bandage). In all cases, a large pad (e.g. of gamgee) should be placed directly beneath the fracture to act as a fulcrum.

37. Thomas splint (g): In long oblique fractures and those with apposition no manipulation will be needed and the traction system may be completed by, for example, tying the cords to the end of the splint (1). The convention of passing the medial cord under the corresponding iron helps to control the tendency to lateral rotation (2). A Chinese windlass (of spatulae or a metal rod) may be used to take up slack (3).

38. Thomas splint (h): Where skeletal traction is being used a metal loop (4) (Tulloch–Brown loop) allows a direct pull to be made in the line of the limb. The loop may be tied to the end of the Thomas splint (5) and tensioned with a windlass as previously described (6). A stirrup (7) may be employed to prevent springing of the loop. Protect the sharp ends of the pin with caps (8).

39. Thomas splint (i): Manipulation: With the exception of the young child, manipulation is advisable if there is loss of bony apposition. With the splint in position, but unattached, an assistant applies strong traction (1) while pressure is applied in the directions deduced from the radiographs (2). When the traction is eased off, the limb remains the same length if a hitch has been obtained (3) but telescopes if not (4).

40. Thomas splint (j): After the traction cords have been attached, the end of the splint can be raised temporarily on a pillow (1) while the limb is bandaged to the splint using, for example, 15 cm (6″) crepe bandages (2). Note, gamgee or wool padding behind the fracture to act as a fulcrum (3), behind the knee to keep it in slight flexion (4), and along the shin to avoid sores (5).

41. Thomas splint (k): The system described is normally referred to as fixed traction in a Thomas splint. The basic principles are straightforward, but it is important that they are thoroughly understood. Muscle tension (mainly quads and hams) tends to produce shortening (1); this can be overcome by traction, for example, through a Steinman pin (2) aided by a loop and traction cord (3). If the traction cord is tied to a ringless Thomas splint, the reduction is maintained so long as a pull is kept on the cord (4); redisplacement occurs if the cord is released (5). This proximal migration is normally prevented by the ring (6) so that the reduction is maintained even when the traction cord is released (7). Note that muscle tone = tension in traction cord = ring pressure.

42. Thomas splint (l): The pressure of the ring of the Thomas splint tends to produce sores (1) (especially in the perineal, groin and ischial tuberosity regions) and must be relieved (3). This is done by applying traction (*c.* 3 kg/8 lb) to the anchored cords (2). If ring pressure is unrelieved, *increase the traction weights.*

43. Thomas splint (m): The traction weights have a tendency to pull the patient down towards the foot of the bed (4). This may continue till the splint comes to rest on the traction pulley (5). This may be countered if it becomes a problem by raising the foot of the bed (6), when the traction weight is balanced by the upward component of the patient's body weight (7).

44. Thomas splint (n): Supporting the limb and the splint (i): To allow the patient to move about the bed and prevent pressure on the heel, it is desirable to support the splint; this may be done most simply by tying a cord from the end of the splint to an overhead bar of the Balkan beam bed. The position of the suspension cord may be adjusted from near the midline to either side. (Illus.: lateral attachment to control external rotation.)

45. Thomas splint (o): Supporting the splint (ii): Some prefer a lively system which can be achieved in various ways, e.g. by weights and a system of pulleys (1). The suspension cord may be arranged in Y-fashion to straddle both irons of the Thomas splint (2). Support for the proximal end of the splint (3) is less clearly an advantage; although often pursued – it may cause extra pressure beneath the ring (4).

46. Thomas splint (p): Supporting the splint (iii): Another form of lively splint support ('the octopus') consists of elastic Bunjee cord (1), which can be adjusted with tensioners (2). The cords are attached to the splint with G-cramps (3) and to cross members of the Balkan beam (4) by means of a bar (5) along which a pulley (6) is free to move, allowing easy movement up and down the bed (7).

47. Thomas splint (q): Check radiographs should be taken after the application of a Thomas splint, after any major adjustment, and thereafter at fortnightly intervals till union.

Corrections: (i) If there is persistent shortening (1) tighten the windlass in a fixed traction system (2). This will inevitably increase ring pressure, and must be compensated by increasing the traction weight (3). (Soft tissue between the bone ends may nevertheless thwart reduction.)

48. Thomas splint (r): Corrections: (ii) Where the proximal fragment is abducted (4) the position may be improved by increasing the traction (5) and abducting the leg (6). The position of the ring traction pulley and the splint supports will require corresponding adjustment. (iii) If the proximal fragment is adducted (7) increase of traction alone (8a) may lead to an improvement in the position. It may be helpful to apply side thrust with a pad (8b) between the leg and the medial side iron. (iv) Flexion and/or abduction of the proximal fragment (9) due to unresisted psoas and gluteal action is frequently a very painful complication. In the young patient, raising the splint (10) and/or abducting the leg and bandaging a local pad in position (11) may bring the fragments into alignment, but this manoeuvre is less certain in the older patient where internal fixation is frequently advisable for femoral fractures at this level and of this type. In any patient in whom this conservative technique is practised, care must be taken to avoid pressure in the region of the anterior superior iliac spine (12).

49. Thomas splint (s): Corrections: (e) Perhaps the commonest residual deformity requiring and amenable to correction is backward sag at the fracture site (13). If a continuous posterior support is used, the padding behind the fracture should be increased in thickness. If separate slings are used, the sling behind the fracture should be tightened and/or the padding behind the fracture increased (14).

50. Thomas splint (t): Aftercare (i): During the first 72 hours following fracture, swelling of the thigh from haematoma and oedema may render the ring tight round its circumference. (Normally it should be easy to put a finger under the ring at any point.) To avoid changing the splint, split the ring with a hacksaw, ease the ends apart, and protect them with adhesive strapping.

51. Thomas splint (u): Aftercare (ii): The following items should be checked daily. Look for impending pressure sores (and take appropriate action). *In the Achilles tendon region* if the slings stop at this level (1); *Under the heel*, if the heel is included (2); If a circular woven support is used, a cruciate incision in it at heel level is prophylactic (3); *Over the malleoli* (4).

54. Thomas splint (x): Aftercare (v): In those cases where skeletal traction is employed, look for:
1. Loosening of the Steinman pin; this may require recentring; other treatment is seldom required, so that traction may be continued.
2. Pin-track infection; a wound swab should be sent for bacteriological examination and the appropriate antibiotic administered. If infection is marked, the traction site may have to be abandoned.
3. Shifting and digging-in of the loop; adjust with padding.

During the period a patient spends in bed he should practise quadriceps and general maintenance exercises. Splintage in children should be continued till union (6–12 weeks). In adults, mobilisation of the knee joint and/or the patient may be possible before union is complete.

52. Thomas splint (v): Aftercare (iii): *The ring area:* Good nursing care is vital to avoid skin breakdown. In addition, for: circumferential tightness, split the ring; perineal pressure, increase the ring traction weight; anterior spine pressure (a), lower the splint (b); pressure below the ring (c), decrease or remove any support weight (d) and place a pillow above the ring (e); pad the edge of the sling if needed (f).

53. Thomas splint (w): Aftercare (iv): Check daily for weakness of ankle dorsiflexion (1) indicative of common peroneal nerve palsy and necessitating careful inspection of the neck of the fibula where the cause is generally felting of the wool padding which then transmits pressure from the side iron (2). Repad, and fit a Sinclair foot support or similar if the palsy is complete: expect recovery in 6 weeks.

55. Early mobilisation techniques (a): Where there is abundant callus and the fracture cannot be sprung, splintage may be discarded and the knee mobilised till there is sufficient mature callus to allow weight bearing.
(b): *The Pearson knee-flexion piece:* this may be used as soon as some stabilising callus appears at the fracture site.
    Method: The traction cord (1) is transferred to the Pearson attachment (2) which is fixed to the Thomas splint (3) and hinges at the level of the knee axis (4). An adjustable cord (5) may be used to gradually advance the range of permissible knee flexion. The end of the Thomas splint is raised (6) and supported (7) while a cord (8) may allow the patient to assist his knee extension manually.

56. Early mobilisation techniques (c): Cast bracing (i): After 4–8 weeks in a Thomas splint, cast bracing may be considered, especially in fractures of the distal half. Many techniques are practised. In a typical procedure the patient is sedated with diazepam, a sandbag placed under the buttocks, and a cast sock drawn over the knee (1). Circular woven bandages (stockingette) encase the limb in two sections (2) and are taped in position (3).

57. Cast bracing (ii): A layer of wool roll is used to protect the bony prominences below the knee (4) and as a single layer of padding in the thigh (5). A below-knee plaster is then applied (6) and completed by turning back and incorporating the circular woven bandage (7). An appropriately sized bucket top of polythene is selected (8), trimmed as required and taped in position (9).

58. Cast bracing (iii): Traction is applied to the leg (10), the bucket is pulled well into the groin (11), a plaster thigh piece applied, moulded in a quadrilateral fashion (to prevent rotation) (12) and completed (13). Maintaining traction in 10° flexion, polycentric hinges (14) are carefully positioned with a jig which is centred on the patella (15). The side-stays (16) are adjusted until the fixation plates (17) lie snugly against the upper and lower plaster components. Large encircling jubilee clips (18) may be used to hold the hinges in position while the jig is removed and flexion function checked. The hinges are plastered in position (19) and a rocker or boot applied (20). The hinges can be unlocked by removal of two set screws (21).

59. Cast bracing (iv): The cast brace affords moderate support of the fracture, and mobilisation of the patient may be commenced – at first using crutches and with the hinges locked. After 1–2 weeks or as progress determines, flexion can be permitted and the crutches gradually discarded. The brace is worn until union is complete.

A number of commercially produced cast-bracing kits are available using materials other than plaster of Paris (e.g. the bucket may be formed from pre-cut plastic sheet which can be temporarily softened by heating and moulded to shape: resin plaster bandages and polyethylene hinges can be employed). In many cases these render the technique comparatively simple, with the result that the so-called weight-relieving calliper, tubed into the patient's shoe, is now much less frequently employed for early mobilisation than it was in the past.

60. Other methods of treating fractures of the femur: Hamilton-Russell traction: This is particularly applicable in the conservative treatment of bilateral fractures; it is a form of balanced traction where the pull on the limb (1) is countered by the body weight (2) through the bed being raised (3). The fracture and distal fragment are supported by a padded canvas sling (4), angled slightly towards the head (5) to counter a tendency to distal drift. The theory behind the classical arrangement is that the line of pull on the femur is the resultant (6) of a parallelogram of forces, where the horizontal component (7) is doubled because of the pulley arrangement (8). Friction losses spoil the theory, and many prefer direct control of all forces (9). This method of treatment, although often useful, gives restricted support to the fracture. Note that balanced traction can be carried out using a Thomas splint bandaged to the limb, but unattached to any of the traction cords.

61. Gallows traction: Children up to the age of 3 years (or 4 if very small and light) are ideally treated by this method, which may sometimes be used at home if the circumstances are suitable. Traction tapes are applied to both legs and fixed to an overhead beam (1) so that the child's buttocks are just clear of the bed (2), making nursing easy. The body weight is responsible for the traction. *Gallows traction should not be used in the older child as there is the risk of vascular spasm and peripheral gangrene.*

62. Hip spica: Stable femoral shaft fractures may be supported by a plaster hip spica (3); this must include the injured leg to the toes, the other leg to above the knee, and extend to above the nipple line ('one and a half hip spica'). A hip spica may be used for the fretful child where good nursing care is available at home (with fortnightly out-patient reviews) or for the badly infected open injury in the adult (see Ch. 11 for application details).

63. Conservative treatment of ipsilateral fracture of the femur and tibia: The complication rate for these combined injuries is high, irrespective of treatment. To allow early mobilisation, internal fixation (e.g. by intramedullary nailing) of both fractures is often preferred. Where conservative treatment is indicated (e.g. in children) a Steinman pin is inserted proximally (1), the tibia manipulated, and a below-knee cast applied incorporating the pin (2). A Thomas splint (3) with traction through the pin (4) controls the femoral fracture.

64. Special situations: (a) Fracture in the confused patient: Where there is a head injury or a senile confusional state, a patient being treated conservatively may try to remove his own splint; it is possible to prevent this by encircling it with plaster bandages laid on top of the normal crepe bandages (Tobruk splint). This procedure may also be used to give extra security when a patient is in transit.

(b) Metastatic fracture: If death is not imminent, intramedullary nailing is advised to relieve pain. Acrylic cement packed round any defect may give sufficient support to allow the patient to bear weight.

(c) Femoral shaft fracture with (acute) ischaemia of the foot: Nearly all will respond to reduction of the fracture which should be carried out under circumstances which will permit exploration should reduction fail. If the femoral artery is in fact divided, compression plating through the exploratory incision will usually give the rigid fixation that is required prior to the vessel reconstruction.

(d) Femoral shaft fracture with nerve palsy: The majority are lesions in continuity, the common peroneal element being most often affected. If there is reason to believe that there may be nerve *division*, exploration and internal fixation may have to be undertaken.

(e) Fracture of the femoral neck and shaft: This combination of injuries must be excluded in every case; note too that the ring of a Thomas splint may obscure the affected area. If the shaft fracture is proximal, both fractures may be treated by dynamic hip screw and long plate, but many prefer a Long Gamma™ 3 nail which is itself the choice in more distal fractures.

(f) Femoral neck fracture with dislocation of the hip: See p. 295.

(g) Fractures of the femoral shaft and patella: Note the following important points: 1. Early mobilisation of the knee is essential for retention of function. 2. Avoid patellar excision when mobilisation of the knee is going to be delayed. 3. Avoid if possible exposure of the femoral fracture and the creation of tethering adhesions between the femur and quadriceps.

The ideal management of this difficult combination of injuries is I-M nailing of the femoral fracture and immediate treatment of the patella appropriate to the type of fracture sustained. If the femoral fracture must be treated conservatively, it is best to leave even badly displaced or comminuted patellar fractures to unite by fibrous union; mobilise the knee as

early as possible; excision of the patella can then be carried out as a late secondary procedure when no further flexion can be gained.

(h) Open fractures: Inspection of the fracture site to exclude intramedullary contamination should be part of the initial debridement. If internal fixation is indicated (especially where there are multiple injuries) the infection rate in Grade I and Grade II injuries is said to be no greater after a meticulous debridement and closed nailing than in closed fractures. Grade IIIA fractures with good skin cover and no medullary contamination can be nailed in reasonable safety if reaming is avoided. Grade III B & C open fractures must be carefully assessed, taking into account the greater risks of infection. In some cases nailing may still be advised, while in others the use of an external fixator may be considered safer. With the latter there is always the risk of pin track infections, and the possibility of infection being spread through the medullary canal if secondary nailing is undertaken. The chances of this occurring seem reduced if replacement nailing can be performed within the first week.

65. Fractures of the femur after hip replacement (a): The Vancouver Classification of these fractures (Duncan and Masri) is well established. Three Groups, some with subdivisions, are recognised: **Type A:** These are the trochanteric fractures (incidence 4%), and are subdivided into A_G and A_L depending on which trochanter is involved. **Type B:** These occur round or just distal to the stem of the prosthesis. In **B1** the prosthesis is stable (incidence 16%).

66. Fractures of the femur after hip replacement (b): Vancouver Classification *ctd:* **Type B2:** Here the prosthesis is unstable (38%). **B3:** The bone stock is inadequate. This is the most serious and hardest to treat (32%). **Type C:** The fracture occurs well below the stem (9%). *Treatment:* **Type A:** If the fracture is stable, conservative management will generally suffice. If the fracture is unstable, then open reduction and internal fixation is generally advised (e.g. with a Dall–Miles cleat and cable grip system).

67. Fractures of the femur after hip replacement (c): *Treatment ctd:* Operative treatment has been advised for all other fractures, generally with bone grafting to encourage union. **B1:** The Dall–Miles system is often recommended. Proximally, cerclage cables are attached to cable sleeves which sit in slots in the plate which is attached to the shaft distally with screws. While additional screws may be inserted obliquely on either side of the prosthetic stem, broaching the original cement mantle is not particularly recommended.

68. Fractures of the femur after hip replacement (d): B2: In this group where there is instability, removal of the original prosthesis and replacement with a long-stemmed device is usually advised. This may require supplementing with cerclage wires or cables, along with routine bone grafting. **B3:** In this most challenging group the treatment of each case must be decided on its merits. Several strategies have been described: 1. The proximal femur may be replaced with an allograft along with a long stemmed prosthesis. This requires supplementation with bone grafting and often cerclage wiring. The patient's own proximal femur may be retained and used as vascularised autograft (by bi-valving it and wrapping it round the allograft). 2. In some cases a less major procedure may be possible; the canal may be cleared of debris, fresh cement inserted taking care to avoid cement extrusion between the fresh fracture surfaces. A plate is then used, with cerclage wiring and screws through the shaft and the new cement mantle. 3. In the older patient, the proximal femur may be resected and replaced with a custom prosthesis (of tumour-replacement type). **C:** Here open reduction and internal fixation are recommended. The selection of the most appropriate fixation device is dependent on the exact site and the particular features of the fracture. These include plates (such as the Liss plate); screw, nail and blade plates; and short cross-pinned intramedullary nails inserted in the retrograde fashion.

69. Supracondylar fractures (Type A fractures of the distal segment – *see Ch. 12/Frame 84 for full AO Classification)* **(a):** In children, fractures in the distal third of the femur are frequently only minimally displaced, and may be successfully treated by the application of a cylinder plaster. Weight bearing should not be permitted till evidence of early union appears on the radiographs, but during this period the patient may be mobilised with crutches.

70. Supracondylar fractures (b): In the adult especially, supracondylar fractures have a strong tendency for the distal fragment to rotate (1) under the continuous pull of the gastrocnemius (2) into a position of posterior angulation (anterior tilting) (3). If these injuries are being treated conservatively, this cannot be controlled by traction in the line of the limb (4). It is necessary to flex the knee and maintain the traction over a fulcrum (5).

71. Supracondylar fractures (c): The necessary degree of knee flexion may be obtained using a Pearson knee flexion piece, or better still by bending the Thomas splint at the level of the fracture (Illus.). Mobilisation of the knee should be started as early as possible, as the risks of knee stiffness from the development of tethering adhesions (between the quadriceps muscle and the fracture) is high.

72. Supracondylar fractures (d): To allow early mobilisation of the knee, internal fixation is to be preferred. Many methods may be employed, including the use of retrograde intramedullary nailing with interlocking screws, LISS plates and locking screws, pre-contoured plates, and a combination dynamic screw and plate (Illus.).

73. Unicondylar fractures (A-O Type B fractures) (a): Where the displacement is slight (Illus.) these injuries may be treated successfully by conservative measures. Traction in a straight Thomas splint may be used for the first 1–2 weeks, but thereafter mobilisation should be started early, either with a Pearson knee-flexion piece or with Hamilton–Russell traction. *Many, however, prefer to treat all fractures of this type by internal fixation.*

74. Unicondylar fractures (b): Certainly if there is a significant displacement with disturbance of the contours of the articular surfaces of the knee, then internal fixation is certainly indicated. Where the bone is of good texture, two cancellous screws (1), with washers (2) to prevent the heads sinking, may be used. A well-contoured buttress plate (3) and cancellous screws or locking screws can be used if the bone is very soft, or where the fracture has occurred in the presence of a knee joint replacement.

75. Unicondylar fractures (c): Shearing fractures which are entirely intra-articular frequently fail to unite if treated conservatively, possibly due to dispersal of the fracture haematoma by the synovial fluid. The resulting non-union is likely to cause knee instability. Fractures of this pattern may be held with two cancellous screws with their heads sunk below the level of the articular surface. Thereafter a 6-week period of non-weight bearing in a motion permitting splint is advised.

76. T- and Y-condylar fractures (A-O Type C fractures) (a): Although undisplaced fractures may be treated conservatively by traction and splintage, internal fixation is generally advised to allow early mobilisation of the knee. Some may be treated with a retrograde I-M nail with interlocking and cancellous screws (Illus.) Ilizarov methods, including hybrid fixation systems may also be employed, and are of especial value where there is gross comminution (e.g. in elderly patients with osteoporotic bone).

77. T- and Y-condylar fractures (b): In high-energy trauma cases bone fragmentation is a characteristic of the primary fracture site, but the extent and area of bone actually involved may not always be obvious on the plain films. This CT scan of what appeared to be a comminuted supracondylar fracture shows a downward extension from the main transverse element, converting it into a T-fracture. In the planned surgical intervention this had to be taken into account.

78. T- and Y-condylar fractures (c): The main fracture was held with a LISS plate and locking screws. The distally placed screws have the double purpose of securing the main distal mass to the contoured end of the plate and preventing widening of the condylar split.

79. T- and Y-condylar fractures (d): 3-D CT scan reconstructions, if available, may offer additional information on the degree of comminution and the orientation of bone fragments. In this example posterior comminution is shown. This is often of considerable benefit in pre-operation planning, and influences the decision as to whether to attempt internal fixation of the fracture or to use, for example, a hybrid or other external fixator. Fixation here in view of the size of the main fragments was by a LISS plate and additional fragment screws.

80. Displaced femoral epiphysis: This injury usually results from hyperextension, and there is risk of vascular complications; reduction should be carried out expeditiously by applying traction, flexing the knee to a right angle and pressing the epiphysis backwards into position. The knee should be kept in flexion for 3 weeks in a plaster slab, and for a further 3–5 weeks in a plaster cylinder in a more neutral position. Alternatively, after reduction the epiphysis may be stabilised with two Kirschner wires across the growth plate.

81. Segmental fractures: These are uncommon in the femur, but are associated with a high incidence of non-union at one level. Fracture exposure may lose the tenuous blood supply to the intermediate segment. Although they may be treated conservatively (dealing with each complication as it arises), closed nailing, if reduction can be accomplished, is a more attractive alternative. A nail, locked at both ends, should be used. Static nailing may be converted at a later stage to dynamic nailing if union is delayed.

82. COMPLICATIONS OF FRACTURES OF THE FEMUR

Among the many complications which may accompany this fracture the following should be noted:

1. Oligaemic shock (see also p. 32): In the presence of multiple injuries there may be concerns about the risks of 'second hit' haemodynamic instability, and the fact that any intramedullary nailing procedure may increase the possibility of embolic fat worsening the pulmonary status; patients with a concomitant chest injury are at particular risk. In greater danger are patients with bilateral femoral fractures, where there is a marked increase in mortality and morbidity. In these circumstances the patient requires very careful assessment, and damage control orthopaedics is often the safest option.

2. Fat embolism (see p. 91)

3. Compartment Syndromes: Involvement of the fascial compartments of the thigh is extremely uncommon because of their large volume and because they blend with those related to the muscles round the hip, allowing extravasation beyond their limits. This complication is seen most often after intramedullary nailing, and the possibility of its occurrence kept in mind. (For details of pressure monitoring and treatment see Ch. 5).

4. Slow or delayed union: These are common complications, and if the fracture is being treated conservatively, may necessitate prolonged immobilisation of the knee, with risk of permanent stiffness.

Where the fracture is being treated by intramedullary nailing, if the nail is not a close fit, undue movement may be occurring at the fracture site; this is particularly likely to be the case in distal fractures. Revision nailing, with reaming (which is said to have an osteogenic effect) and the insertion of a wider nail usually result in union.

Where a locked intramedullary nail is used, conversion from static to dynamic locking (by removal of the appropriate interlocking screws) may encourage union.

5. Non-union: In fractures being treated conservatively, this is generally dealt with as soon as it is confidently diagnosed, by intramedullary nailing and bone grafting.

If non-union occurs in a fracture which has been treated by intramedullary nailing, bone grafting will also usually be required. In addition, the quality of the fixation must be reviewed, and if this is found wanting, it must be dealt with. In some cases this will involve replacing the nail (after reaming the canal) with one of a larger diameter. Rotational instability must be controlled, and the use of interlocking screws is desirable. In some cases, in order to obtain compression of the fragments, the use of a dynamic compression plate may be considered.

6. Mal-union: In conservatively treated fractures persistent lateral angulation is the commonest deformity, and if 25° or more then correction by osteotomy and intramedullary nailing should be considered. Anterior or posterior angulation seldom gives rise to much difficulty. Nearer the knee, angulation showing on the AP radiographs may give rise to instability, difficulty in walking and secondary osteoarthritis of the knee. Each case must be assessed on its own merits, but again corrective osteotomy/osteoclasis should be considered.

Where intramedullary nailing has been carried out, angulation showing on the AP or lateral projections is seldom a problem in mid-shaft fractures unless there has been failure of the fixation device. Moderate and usually acceptable angulation in these planes may occur in distal third fractures.

Rotational deformity in cases treated by intramedullary nailing may require correction. If recognised when the fracture is still mobile, this may be dealt with by revision of the placement of the interlocking screws. If union has occurred, a rotational osteotomy may be performed and maintained with a reamed interlocking intramedullary nail.

7. Limb shortening: Moderate shortening in the adult should be corrected by shoe alteration to within 1–2 cm (½″) of the limb discrepancy. In the carefully selected, more severe case, lengthening may be considered using a modified Ilizarov technique over an intramedullary nail.

In children, any difference in leg length usually corrects (or indeed overcorrects) spontaneously within 6–18 months of the injury, and alteration to the shoes is seldom required. Only rarely in epiphyseal injuries is there progressive shortening.

8. Knee stiffness: This is a common complication of femoral and tibial fractures, and of injuries to the extensor mechanism of the knee. Among the factors which are involved are the following:

(a) *Quadriceps tethering:* If the quadriceps becomes adherent to a femoral shaft fracture, it becomes unable to glide over the smooth distal shaft in the normal fashion. This results in fixation of the patella and restriction of movement in the knee. The closer the fracture is to the knee, the more important is this effect. Surgical intervention tends to aggravate this tendency and manipulation under anaesthetic may not be effective unless they can be followed by rapid mobilisation. Some advocate the use of a continuous passive motion machine in the immediate postoperative period, with either an epidural or a nerve block for pain relief.

(b) *Fractures involving the knee joint:* Fractures which involve the articular surfaces may give rise to intra-articular and periarticular adhesions, or may form a mechanical block to movement. Early mobilisation is especially desirable where a fracture involves the joint, and the use of continuous passive motion equipment is often advocated.

(c) *Prolonged immobilisation:* Fixation of the knee for an undesirably long period, for example, by delay in union, may lead to stiffness, and this effect is particularly marked in the elderly.

9. Infection: Infection may sometimes supervene in femoral shaft fractures treated by intramedullary nailing. Sometimes the source is obvious (e.g. from a contaminated open wound where the initial debridement has been unsuccessful or insufficiently scrupulous), but often it may unaccountably follow a meticulously performed closed procedure. The course of treatment must be individually determined, but the following guidelines usually apply:

1. The causal organism should be isolated, and the appropriate antibiotic administered in effective doses for an adequate length of time.

2. If the infection has become established, it is unlikely to respond unless the fracture is firmly supported, and a most thorough debridement carried out under antibiotic cover.

3. If the fixation afforded by the nail remains good, the nail may be retained, but here as in those cases where the fixation is poor, removal of the nail is

often advocated. At the time of the debridement and after removal of the nail, the canal may be reamed to permit the (later) insertion of a larger (by 2–2.5 mm in diameter) nail, and irrigated thoroughly with 10 L of saline; a drainage hole placed in the distal femoral cortex facilitates the fluid flow. The limb is placed in traction or an external fixator applied. Intravenous antibiotics are administered. A repeat debridement may be required in 48 hours. If negative post debridement cultures are obtained then repeat nailing may then be performed; if not, then it will be necessary to continue with an external fixator although it may be difficult to maintain a good hold on the fracture as Schanz pins in the metaphysis have a tendency to loosen.

AFTERCARE

1. Immediate post-operative: See Frame 21.

2. Quadriceps exercises: Stability in the knee and extension power are dependent on a good quadriceps. It is important that the muscle is not allowed to waste, and quadriceps exercises should be started as soon after the injury as possible, and intensified on removal of any fixation. (Amongst the few exceptions are injuries to the extensor mechanism where quadriceps exercises are usually delayed for 2 weeks in case early contraction endangers a repair.)

3. Flexion exercises: These should also be commenced as soon as possible, provided the means can be devised to support the fracture fully. Flexion should not be permitted unless stress on the fracture can be reduced to a safe level or where healing can be more or less guaranteed (e.g. tibial plateau fractures).

4. Discarding walking aids: Walking without the support of sticks or crutches is frequently followed by an improvement in flexion, and such supportive measures should be discontinued as soon as the state of union and the patient's balance will allow.

5. Physiotherapy: Ideally quadriceps and flexion exercises should be supervised by a physiotherapist with access to aids and facilities such as weights, slings, local heat and hydrotherapy, but basically the patient should be instructed in quadriceps and flexion exercises, and the importance of performing these frequently should be stressed. Passive mobilisation of the patella in appropriate cases may also be helpful.

Physiotherapy should be continued until an acceptable functional range has been achieved (see below) or until a static position has been reached. For this it is necessary to record the range of movements in the knee with accuracy; this should be done initially at weekly and then at monthly intervals. A measurable gain in range, no matter how small, is an encouragement to the patient to further effort; and on the other hand the absence of any improvement should make it clear to him that to continue treatment is not justifiable.

In routine cases treated by intramedullary nailing, recovery of a full range of flexion is achieved in the majority of cases in 12 months, with most of the gain occurring in the first 3 months.

NOTES

Acceptable functional range What is acceptable obviously varies considerably from case to case, being dependent on the gravity of the injury, the age of the patient, his occupation, athletic or outdoor pursuits, hobbies, etc., but the basic aim is a stable knee which places little restraint on normal everyday activities. The following factors are important.

Lack of extension Loss of extension, both active and passive, may be found, e.g. in an angulated supracondylar fracture of the femur, or where there has been previous osteoarthritis in the knee. Such losses are seldom severe enough to cause appreciable disability, usually being compensated at hip and ankle. If the knee can be passively but not actively extended, this is known as an *extension lag*. Extension lag frequently gives rise to 'giving way' of the knee. It is common to some degree after most cases where a patellectomy has been performed, but usually recovers if quadriceps exercises are intensified.

Where extension lag is due to quadriceps tethering, quadriceps exercises should also be encouraged. The patient in most cases of persistent lag learns to compensate for the disability by using the hip extensors to keep the knee straight while standing.

Lack of flexion Appreciable disability follows if flexion to 100° (i.e. 10° more than right-angle flexion) cannot be obtained, and 100° should be the aim. Flexion to 80–90° will permit sitting in inside seats (i.e. non-aisle seats) in public transport, cinemas, etc., but will not allow the patient to kneel. Less than 100° will cause difficulty with steps, deep tread and narrow stairs, and if both knees are affected, rising from armless chairs.

Where flexion has just become static at less than 100°, manipulation of the knee under general anaesthesia should be considered. This is best avoided, however, after patellectomy and quadriceps tendon and patellar ligament repairs because of the risks of secondary rupture. Gains in flexion by manipulation are seldom high, and late manipulations are usually very unrewarding. Arthroscopy should be considered, with division of any intra-articular adhesions.

Where 80° or less flexion is possible and the position static, the patient's functional disability and functional requirements should be carefully assessed. If there is a marked deficit, quadricepsplasty should be considered. In this procedure the vasti are divided close to the knee so that their tethering effect is eliminated; rectus femoris then becomes the sole extensor of the knee. This often gives a useful gain (often in the region of 40°) although sometimes this is at the expense of an extension lag, and always with some loss of power.

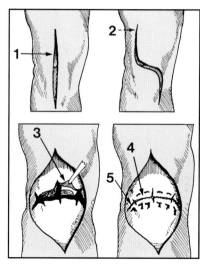

95. Treatment (a): If the joint surface can be restored, the fragments may be held by AO tension band wiring: two hooked Kirschner wires (1) are inserted, round which is looped a wire (2) tightened by twisting. A second wire in a figure-of-eight (3) may be used (as may a figure-of-eight with the inferior limb in a hole drilled through the patella). The K wires are sunk home (4) and trimmed (5). *Pyrford wiring* which uses a wire loop (6) and purse string (7) is strong, but is not advised because of the risks of avascular necrosis of the patella.

96. Treatment (b): If the joint surfaces cannot be restored and held, or if as illustrated, there is much fragmentation, a complete patellar excision should be carried out, with repair of the quadriceps insertion and lateral expansions (which are invariably damaged). Note, however, that if the damage is confined to one pole of the patella, and the major part of the patella is spared, then good results can be obtained by *partial patellectomy*.

97. Treatment (c): For exploration or excision, the patella may be exposed through a midline vertical incision (best where further surgery is required) (1) or a lazy S (2) with the raising of two flaps. The patellar fragments are carefully dissected free, taking care that every piece is removed (3). The insertion (4) along with the lateral expansions (5) are repaired with mattress sutures and a plaster cylinder applied. Crutches should be used for 4 weeks and mobilisation commenced at 6 weeks.

98. Avulsion fractures of the tibial tubercle: In the adult, or adolescent near skeletal maturity (Illus.) the displacement, if marked, should be reduced and the tubercle fixed with a screw. If displacement is slight, a 6-week period in a plaster cylinder should suffice. In children, surgery should be avoided if possible because of the risks of premature epiphyseal fusion but, if manipulative reduction fails, open reduction and fixing with a suture may become necessary.

99. Rupture of the quadriceps tendon: The diagnosis is essentially clinical; it may sometimes be suggested by examination of the soft-tissue shadows on the radiographs (Illus.), by ultrasound, or MRI scan. The tendon must be re-attached surgically; and it is often necessary to drill the patella to provide anchorage for the sutures. Thereafter a plaster cylinder is applied. Quadriceps exercises are commenced at 2 weeks, weight bearing at 4 weeks and knee flexion at 6 weeks.

100. Rupture of the patellar ligament: Radiographs show proximal displacement of the patella (Illus.); ultrasound or MRI scans may be helpful. Repair the tendon, using a tension relieving wire suture (for 6 weeks) between the patella and tibial tubercle. Avulsions of the distal tip of the patella may be treated by excision and re-attachment of the ligament (using holes drilled through the patella and a tension relieving wire), but better results are claimed[1] fixing the fragment to the patella with a metal basket and screws.

101. Osgood Schlatter's disease: In children, sudden or repeated quadriceps contraction may be responsible for this condition, which is characterised by recurrent pain, tenderness, and swelling over the tibial tubercle. It may be mistaken for an acute injury. While slow spontaneous resolution is the rule, an acute episode may be treated by 2 weeks in a plaster cylinder. Severe persistent symptoms occasionally merit excision of the detached fragment.

102. Acute lateral dislocation of the patella (a): The patella dislocates laterally, often due to a sudden muscular contraction or a blow on its medial side. It may be reduced by firm lateral pressure (anaesthesia is seldom required). A 6-week period in a cast is advised for a first incident. An MRI scan is invaluable in showing any associated chondral injury. Some advise early arthroscopy, washing out blood and any loose bodies, re-attaching any large osteochondral fragment, and early mobilisation.

103. Patellar dislocation (b): Lateral dislocation commonly occurs as a first or subsequent incident in the course of recurrent dislocation of the patella, a condition seen most frequently in teenage girls. The presence on the tangential projection of the knee of a marginal osteochondral fracture is diagnostic, but may not be obvious until some weeks after a first incident (which may also be overlooked if spontaneous reduction occurs).

104. Patellar dislocation (c): As the femur meets the tibia at an angle, the quadriceps (1) and patellar ligament (2) have a *lateral component* (3) during muscle contraction; this is greater where there is genu valgum (5); it is resisted by the femoral gutter (4). An error in tracking may cause the patella to dislocate. When this *starts in extension*, patella alta (6) or an abnormal quadriceps insertion (8) may be factors. In these particular cases a re-alignment procedure may be required (e.g. Elmslie–Trillat, Hauser (9) or Galeazzi); in the latter, more suitable in the adolescent, the divided semitendinosus tendon is threaded through a hole in the patella (10), and the stump sewn to semimembranosus (11). Where the dislocation occurs *in flexion* there may be hypoplasia of the patella or lateral femoral condyle (7), with a shallow sulcus and tilting of the patella. Such cases may respond to a lateral tissue (vastus lateralis) release, with or without medial reefing, but they may also require a re-alignment procedure. If there is no tracking problem, ligament laxity is sometimes blamed. Many respond to physiotherapy (concentrating on the oblique fibres of vastus medialis) and the use of a knee brace during athletic activities.

105. Dislocation of the knee (a): This generally follows a major traumatic episode, although surprisingly, it may sometimes result from comparatively minor trauma. Most commonly the tibia is displaced anteriorly, but medial, lateral, posterior and rotational displacements are also found. There is inevitably major damage to the ligaments of the knee; all or most may be torn along with the joint capsule. Note that clinical examination has been shown to give a more accurate assessment of ligamentous damage than MRI scanning.

106. Dislocation of the knee (b): Sometimes there is displacement of the menisci, fractures of the tibial spines, common peroneal nerve palsy, and most seriously, popliteal artery damage. Initial investigations should include plain films and an MRI scan. *Treatment:* Closed reduction should be carried out as expeditiously as possible. Reduction is generally easy with traction and the application of pressure over the displaced tibia. Then, in most cases, arteriography is advised, followed if required by popliteal artery exploration. Surgery is also indicated if closed reduction fails (generally due to button-holing of the capsule by a femoral condyle) or if there is a common peroneal nerve palsy.

The soft tissue injuries may be dealt with surgically or conservatively, with the best results claimed for the former if carried out within the first 3 weeks. A careful assessment of the extent of the injury is mandatory, based on the preoperative findings, examination of the knee under anaesthesia for the degree of ligamentous laxity, and arthroscopy. Harner et al[2] advise that any cruciate ligament reconstructions be performed first, and under a tourniquet; this should be followed by direct repair of torn collateral ligaments after release of the tourniquet; the menisci should be preserved wherever possible. Postoperatively a brace is worn for 6 weeks, with the first 4 weeks with it locked in extension. Intense quadriceps exercise are practised from the outset, and passive flexion started at 4 weeks.

In the conservative management of these cases, where surprisingly, good results preponderate, the leg should be supported after reduction by light traction (2–3 kg/6 lb) in a Thomas splint for 3–4 weeks; this may be followed by a further 4 weeks in a plaster cylinder before mobilisation is commenced.

107. Soft-tissue injuries of the knee: When there has been trauma to the knee and the radiographs show little in the way of bony injury, the possibility of a significant soft-tissue injury should be considered. It would be unrealistic to say that injuries of this type are easy to diagnose; they sometimes are, but often cause much difficulty. There is the common clinical picture of pain in the knee, swelling, and difficulty in weight bearing shared by many lesions. Investigation of each case should aim firstly to localise the injury to a specific structure, although it must be accepted that localising tenderness may be difficult to ascertain where there has been an associated fracture in the region. An attempt should be made to exclude the following:
1. Damage to the extensor apparatus
2. Lateral dislocation of the patella with spontaneous reduction
3. Tears of the ligaments of the knee
4. Meniscus tears.

In some centres, when the injury is suspected of being more than trivial, further investigation is pursued in an aggressive fashion: any haemarthrosis is aspirated, and the soft-tissue elements examined by MRI scan and/or arthroscopy. Note that the presence of a substantial haemarthrosis is generally associated with damage to a major structural element. Aspiration is usually required to permit a more meaningful examination, and general anaesthesia is advisable. Any suggestion of locking or other evidence of meniscal damage merits further investigation by arthroscopy or MRI scan (because if a meniscus is torn and suitable for surgical repair, this is best undertaken within 4 weeks of the injury).

If there is no hard evidence to implicate any of the major soft tissue structures (and this is so in the *majority* of cases) a provisional (and rather unsatisfactory) diagnosis of 'knee sprain' or 'sprained ligaments with traumatic effusion' may be made, and the case treated appropriately (e.g. by the application of a crepe bandage support, Jones pressure bandage, or circular woven bandage (Tubigrip®)). The case should be re-assessed at weekly intervals thereafter until either the symptoms have settled completely, or a more accurate diagnosis can be established.

108. Medial ligament injuries (a): The commonest cause is a blow on the lateral side of the knee (1) which forces the joint into valgus (2). With slight force, there is partial tearing of the medial ligament (knee sprain) and the knee remains stable on clinical testing. With greater violence, the deep portion of the ligament ruptures (partial tear) (3); stressing the knee in 30° flexion with the foot internally rotated (F) causes more opening up of the joint than normal, but stressing the joint in extension (E) has no effect. There may be clinical evidence of rotatory instability. With greater violence, superficial *and* deep parts of the ligament rupture (4) and the tear rapidly spreads across the posterior ligament (5). The medial meniscus (6) may also tear. When the knee is stressed in extension (E) slight to moderate opening up will be noted, and if the edge of the ligament rolls over it may be felt subcutaneously (7). With severe violence, the cruciates (especially the anterior cruciate) rupture (8) and the joint opens widely on stressing as at (E). Bruising on the lateral side (9) and medial tenderness (10) are suggestive of medial ligament damage. If there is remaining doubt regarding its integrity, repeat clinical tests after aspiration, or take stress radiographs, comparing one side with the other.

109. Medial ligament injuries (b): Treatment:
(i) Sprain: Crepe bandages or a Jones pressure bandage should be applied and the patient given crutches to use until the acute symptoms have settled: review at least twice.
(ii) Isolated tear, with no evidence of 'rolling over' of the medial ligament: POP fixation *with the knee at 45° flexion* for 8 weeks, or the use of a limited motion (30–60°) knee brace. Review at 1 week to exclude associated meniscal injury.
(iii) Major tear: If isolated and uncomplicated, conservative management may be pursued (e.g. with a limited motion brace), and a good result expected. If under anaesthesia gross instability is found, this is suggestive of posterior capsular tearing and/or involvement of other major structures. Exploration and repair of the medial ligament and posteromedial capsule are then advised. An associated meniscus injury should be carefully assessed and treated on its merits: the meniscus should be preserved if feasible, and in some cases it may be possible to re-attach or repair it. If the anterior cruciate ligament has been detached or torn, it may be re-attached or repaired, or this deferred until later when knee movements have been regained.

Complications of medial ligament injury:
(a) Late valgus instability: It may be possible to improve stability by a reconstructive procedure; semitendinosus may be rerouted and used to reinforce a defective medial ligament, or a prosthetic ligament replacement may be carried out.

(b) Persistent rotatory instability: Improvement may follow a medial capsular repair and pes anserinus transposition, although the late results are often disappointing.

110. Pelligrini–Stieda disease: A valgus strain of the knee may produce partial avulsion of the medial ligament, with subsequent calcification in the subperiosteal haematoma. There is prolonged pain and local tenderness, with limitation of flexion, but no instability. In the acute phase, plaster immobilisation for 2–3 weeks is advised, followed by mobilisation. Local hydrocortisone infiltrations are sometimes advocated for the chronic case.

111. Injuries to the lateral ligament (a): The lateral ligament (1) is part of a complex which includes the biceps femoris tendon (2) and the fascia lata (3) attached to tibia, fibula and patella. All these structures may be damaged if the knee is subjected to a varus stress (4), and with severe violence the cruciates (5) will also be torn. The common peroneal nerve (6) may be stretched or torn.

112. Lateral ligament (b): Test the stability of the knee by applying a varus stress with the knee in extension (1), looking for opening-up of the joint on the lateral side (2). Test for common peroneal involvement by looking for weakness of dorsiflexion of the foot and toes (3), and/or sensory loss on the dorsum of the foot and side of the leg (4).

113. Lateral ligament (c): In some cases the radiographs may show tell-tale avulsion fractures of the fibular head or tibia. (Illus.: note a small undisplaced fracture of the head of the fibula produced by the lateral ligament (the fracture highlighted with black arrows), and a large displaced fragment, (indicated with white arrows) avulsed by the biceps.) *Treatment:* 1. If the knee is clinically stable, symptomatic treatment only is required (e.g. a crepe bandage and crutches).

114. Lateral ligament: Treatment *ctd:*
2. If there is instability, operative repair of the ligament and repair of the posterolateral capsule (if involved) is indicated, unless there is a definite, undisplaced fracture which seems likely to go on to union; in such circumstances a plaster cylinder should be applied and retained for 6–8 weeks before mobilisation.
3. Common peroneal nerve palsy, if present, is likely to be due either to a lesion in continuity, or a complete disruption of the nerve over an extensive area. If the ligament is being repaired, the opportunity should be taken to inspect the nerve. (Some advocate exploration of the nerve in all cases, irrespective of the need for repair of the lateral ligament, holding the view that this gives the opportunity of carrying out a local decompression should this be required, and thereby perhaps aiding recovery.) In all cases treatment for drop foot should be started. With a lesion in continuity, recovery usually starts within 6 weeks, but a disruptive lesion carries a poor prognosis.

148. Describe this fracture: how is it being treated? Assuming conservative treatment was being continued, would you make any correction?

149. What does the radiograph show? What structure is at serious risk?

150. What is this fracture? How has it been treated? What alternative treatment might have been carried out?

151. What does this 3-D reconstruction show? How might this be treated?

152. What two distinct fractures does this radiograph show? How might they be treated?

ANSWERS TO SELF-TEST

138. Proximal third fracture of the femur being treated in a Thomas splint. The proximal fragment is flexed so that there is no bony apposition, and probably soft tissue between the bone ends. The position is unacceptable (risk of non-union or mal-union) and internal fixation would be advocated. (AO = 32–A3.1)

139. Oblique fracture of the midshaft of the femur (with shortening and angulation) in a child. It is being treated in a plaster hip spica. The position is acceptable: union is likely to be rapid; the shortening will almost certainly resolve spontaneously; any residual angulation is also likely to disappear with re-modelling. (AO = 32–A2.2)

140. Supracondylar fracture of the femur. Angulation is slight, and is in the reverse direction from normal. Traction in a straight Thomas splint might be used and mobilisation commenced at an early date. Alternatively, this fracture might be dealt with by Hamilton–Russell traction and cast bracing or internal fixation with a blade plate, a dynamic condylar screw or an intramedullary nail with interlocking screws. (AO = 33–A1.2)

141. There is a fracture of the midshaft of the femur and a supracondylar fracture, both held in alignment with an intramedullary nail. In addition, there is a fracture of the proximal third of the tibia. Such injuries are typical of high-velocity road traffic accidents. (AO = 32–B1.2 + (33–A2.3 or 32–B2.3) + 41–A3)

142. Fracture of the femoral shaft at the level of the tip of a replacement arthroplasty prosthesis (Type B1 fracture). Treat by open reduction and internal fixation, e.g. using a plate and cerclage wiring (such as the Dall-Miles system).

143. Displaced, intra-articular fracture of the medial femoral condyle. Treat by open reduction and internal fixation with counter-sunk cancellous bone screws; otherwise non-union is likely even if reduction is achieved. Avascular necrosis of the fragment is probable. Were the fragment larger, a buttress plate would be considered. (AO = 33–B2.2)

144. Highly comminuted fracture of the distal third of the femur, with a fracture extending between the femoral condyles. Surgical reconstruction is likely to prove difficult due to the degree of comminution, but might be attempted using, for example, the Liss plate system with locking screws or a precontoured plate. Alternatively, conservative management with traction and early mobilisation should be considered. (AO = 33–C3.3)

145. Fracture of the midshaft of the femur, treated by intramedullary nailing. Union is incomplete and the nail has bent, with angulation of the femur because of premature weight bearing. The nail should be removed without delay, and a new nail substituted after reaming. Removal of the nail will obviously be difficult. It may be possible to straighten the bend by forcible manipulation, but if this fails it may be necessary to expose the fracture, saw through the nail and extract the two fragments separately. (AO = 32–A3.2)

146. Supracondylar fracture of the femur supported with a one-piece blade plate and screws. (AO = 32–A3.3)

147. Highly comminuted fracture of the distal portion of the patella, with retraction of the main fragment. The proportion of the patellar surface involved and the degree of comminution militates against preservation, but a final decision should be postponed until the fracture has been thoroughly assessed on exposure. Options include re-attachment with a basket or excision with repair of the ruptured lateral expansions.

148. Fracture of the femoral shaft at the junction between the middle and distal thirds, with posterior angulation (anterior tilting of the distal fragment). It is being treated in a Thomas splint (note the side iron). Traction should be increased, and further padding placed under the fracture to correct the angulation. (AO = 32–A2.2)

149. Dislocation of the knee (posterior dislocation with 90° rotational deformity superimposed). The popliteal artery, in particular, is in grave danger.

150. A transverse fracture has been anatomically reduced and held with a single cortical screw. This method of fixation is prone to failure due to the magnitude of the distracting forces. A tension band wiring system is to be preferred.

151. There is a fracture of the lateral tibial plateau and the neck of the fibula, with an associated transverse fracture of the tibia close to the metaphyso-diaphyseal junction. Although such an injury might be treated conservatively, internal fixation allows early mobilisation and decreases the risks of knee stiffness. In this case a PERILOC™ plate was used with locked screws. Note the clustering of the skin clips which indicate that the device was inserted using minimally invasive techniques through three separate incisions.

152. 1. There has been a Schatzker type II fracture of the lateral tibial plateau. Due to the displacement, open reduction and internal fixation are desirable, and here this has been achieved using screws. A buttress plate may also be used in this situation.

2. There has been an avulsion of the proximal attachment of the patellar ligament. It is desirable to preserve the patella and re-attach the ligament. Here this was done using drill holes through the patella to provide suture anchorage. A quadrilateral wire through the patella and tibial tubercle has been placed to relieve strain in the sutures. This would be retained for 6 weeks.

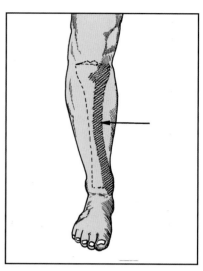

1. General principles (a): Mechanisms of injury: The tibia is vulnerable to torsional stresses (1) (e.g. sporting injuries), to violence transmitted through the feet (2) (e.g. falls from a height, road traffic accidents), and from direct blows (3) (e.g. road traffic accidents, blows from falling rock, masonry, etc.).

2. General principles (b): Isolated fractures of either the tibia or fibula may occur from direct violence (1) although this is comparatively uncommon. As in the case of the forearm bones, indirect violence leads to fracture of both tibia and fibula (2). Always obtain radiographs of the whole length of the limb to exclude a distal injury accompanying a proximal fracture (3).

3. General principles (c): Note that a third of the tibia is subcutaneous. There is little to resist the spiky end of a fractured tibia from penetrating the skin; again, any direct violence to the shin is uncushioned, and the skin is readily split; these factors account for the fact that tibial fractures are often open (either from within out or from without in).

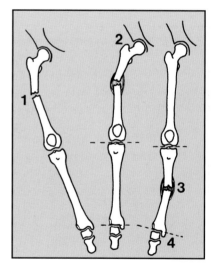

4. General principles (d): Partly because of its triangular shape, and partly because of the frequency of injury caused by torsional forces, oblique and spiral fractures of the tibia are common. Muscle tone in the soleus (1), gastrocnemius (2) and tibialis anterior (3) tends to produce shortening and displacement in fractures of this type (4).

5. General principles (e): The popliteal artery (5) is anchored as it passes under the origin of the soleus at the soleal line (6). It is susceptible to damage in upper tibial fractures (7) and may cause Volkmann's ischaemia of the calf with permanent flexion contracture of the ankle. Fractures of the tibia may be followed by ischaemia of the distal fragment (8) through interruption of the blood supply through the nutrient artery (9).

6. General principles (f): It is particularly important to correct angulation in fractures of this weight-bearing bone. Unlike angulation in femoral shaft fractures (1), which can be compensated at the hip (2), residual angulation in tibial fractures (3) will throw inevitable stress at the ankle (4) and/or the knee, perhaps leading to pain and secondary osteoarthritis.

51. Special situations (c): In some cases of high-energy trauma both the shaft and metaphysis are involved. The degree of metaphyseal involvement prevents the use of the pins of a fixator being inserted proximally. In these circumstances it may be possible to use a hybrid apparatus: proximally wires through the metaphysis are held under tension in a ring; this is then connected by a system of rods and traction pins to the distal fragment, offering the possibilities of applying traction and adjusting the relative positions of the proximal and distal elements.

In the case illustrated, note the segmental fracture of the tibial diaphysis with a large central fragment; the fracture of the fibula at the level of the mid and distal thirds; and the highly comminuted fracture of the metaphysis extending into the knee joint.

Rings with tension wires have been inserted proximally and distally, with an additional threaded distal pin. The linkage in this case is the Taylor Spacial System which permits very precise control over the relative position of the various elements. Note the restoration of excellent alignment and length.

52. Special situations (d): Fractures of the distal shaft: Many can be treated conservatively by reduction and plaster fixation, with or without a Steinman pin through the heel to help maintain alignment; but some restriction of ankle joint movements is common. Alternatively, a number of methods of internal fixation, allowing early movements, may be used. These include PERI-LOC™ plates with locking screws, intramedullary nails with cross screws, and a fine-wire/Steinman pin hybrid fixator system. (See also plafond fractures p. 397.)

53. Special situations (e): Isolated fractures of the fibula: The fibula may be fractured by direct violence; symptomatic treatment only is required (e.g. a below-knee walking plaster for 6 weeks). Always ensure, however, that the tibia is not fractured at another level, or that the fibular fracture represents part of a more complex injury to the ankle joint.

54. Special situations (f): Severely displaced fractures in children: While the majority of these may be managed conservatively as previously described, other methods are available. These include the use of flexible intramedullary nails. (In the case illustrated of a tibial fracture at the junction of the middle and distal thirds, three nails have been used, inserted from above. Other methods include the use of an external fixator (with 2 pins on each side of the fracture), and plating).

55. SPECIAL SITUATIONS (g): OPEN FRACTURES

The frequency with which fractures of the tibia are found to be open, and the reasons for this have been given at the beginning of this section. The AO and Gustilo classifications of open fractures, are dealt with separately in Chapter 1; some general guidelines in the management of open fractures (including skin replacement methods) are commented upon in Chapter 3. In this common fracture situation some additional details may require consideration.

INITIAL TREATMENT

1. The limb should be re-aligned if there is gross deformity.
2. The state of the peripheral pulses should be documented. If absent and not restored by re-alignment, there may be need for arteriography.
3. Note if there is absence of sensation in the foot; such a finding may be important if amputation needs to be considered.
4. Document the location and dimensions of the wounds. Remove any gross contaminants (such as grass or leaves). Make a photographic record of the wounds (e.g. using a Polaroid camera or a digital camera with a print out) to avoid any further disturbance before the case is taken to theatre.
5. Take a bacteriological swab and commence antibiotics. (For Gram +ve organisms in all cases; in addition, for Gram -ve organisms where there is gross contamination; in addition, for anaerobes if there is contamination with soil, river or lake water). If the patient has received tetanus protection within the previous 5 years, no further preventative measures need be taken. If the protection was given over 5 years previously, then booster prophylaxis should be administered. If there has never been any tetanus protection or this is doubtful, then give toxoid along with tetanus immune globulin.
6. Seal the wounds with a sterile dressing.
7. If there is likely to be any problem with skin cover, then consultation with an experienced plastic surgeon is advised at this stage.

TREATMENT IN THEATRE

1. The wound(s) should be extended to allow a thorough inspection of all possible soiled tissue, including the fractured bone ends. Any wound extension should follow the so-called safe incisions (see p. 375).
2. Non-viable skin should be excised until good dermal bleeding is found. If in doubt, especially over the anterior border of the tibia, leave any doubtful skin until the second inspection.
3. Excise any dead muscle. If there is doubt (and this is often the case), this should also be left until the second inspection.
4. In the case of bone, ideally all devitalised separate fragments should be removed, but any major articular segments (e.g. of the tibial plateau) should be retained; otherwise retention of completely free segments should be only rarely considered because of the much higher rate of infection.
5. Perform a prophylactic fasciotomy on any muscle compartment directly involved, and consider fasciotomies of the remaining compartments if the injury has been a high-energy one.
6. Carry out a thorough lavage, preferably using a pulsatile system, with up to 10L of saline.

7. If contamination has been great, the use of antibiotic beads should be considered.

8. The original wounds should always be left open (although good results following primary closure have been claimed in children where contamination has been minimal). Closure of any wound extension is often permissible at this stage. In many cases the use of vacuum dressings may be helpful in providing better quality drainage, reducing oedema and minimising wound size, and stimulating healing by increasing local blood flow.

FIXATION OF THE FRACTURE

There has been much controversy over the use of internal fixation in the treatment of open fractures, but in many cases the fears expressed of increasing the risks of infection have been shown to be unjustified. In open fractures of Types 1 & 2 (Gustilo) the infection rate following intramedullary nailing using the closed technique has been shown to be low, and no greater than in closed injuries of a similar pattern.

In Grade 3 open fracture it has been suggested that reaming of the medullary cavity is undesirable, and for this reason a solid intramedullary nail is often advocated. The nail chosen must be of sufficiently small diameter to allow it to negotiate the tibial canal without sticking, and if made of titanium should still prove of adequate strength. Others have shown that in the majority of Grade 3 open fractures that the results of nailing (with the use of locking screws) after reaming are comparable in terms of infection with those obtained where external fixators have been employed; and that they are better in terms of joint stiffness, mal-union, access for plastic reconstructions, and patient preference. Nevertheless, where there has been gross tissue contamination, many would still prefer to use an external fixator or where applicable, a simple plaster cast support until the situation regarding wound infection has been resolved.

SECOND INSPECTION

This should be performed about 48 hours after the primary procedure. Any necrotic tissue should be excised and irrigation repeated. Further inspections are dictated by the findings at this stage. Once the soft tissue bed is stable, secondary wound closure may be carried out. If any plastic surgical procedure (such as a fasciocutaneous flap, see p. 71) is going to be needed, the aim should be to get the tissue bed in a state suitable for this by the fifth day, as this greatly increases the chances of success. Split skin grafting is not suitable for bone which has no periosteal cover, or tendon without paratenon. The following techniques have been recommended for consideration in open fractures with substantial skin defects:

Proximal third
- Proximally based medial or lateral fasciocutaneous flap.
- Gastrocnemius muscle flap.
- Free flap.

Middle third
- Proximally or distally based, medial or lateral fasciocutaneous flap.
- Anterior compartment muscle flap.
- Soleus muscle flap.
- Free flap.

Distal third
- Distally based fasciocutaneous flap.
- Free flap.

Ankle
- Free flap.

Note also the following:
1. If at inspection there is no indication of infection, an external fixator may be replaced with an intramedullary nail; provided this is done within the first week, the risks of infection are slight. If, however, there is at any time a pin track infection following the use of an external fixator, reaming of the medullary canal is contraindicated as it carries the almost certain risk of disseminating infection throughout the bone.
2. If there is a bone defect involving more than 50% of the circumference of the bone, and more than 2cm long, then bone grafting will ultimately be required in all cases; where the bone defect is smaller, healing may occur without grafting.

56. DIAGNOSIS AND TREATMENT OF COMPARTMENT SYNDROMES

This complication is seen most frequently associated with severe soft tissue damage, especially in high-energy trauma. It is said to occur more frequently after intramedullary nailing, especially where reaming has been carried out, or after prolonged excessive traction. It is not confined to closed fractures. Close observation is required in all these circumstances, and if treatment is delayed for more than 6 hours there will usually be some permanent damage.

DIAGNOSIS

The first symptoms are of severe or increasing pain or tightness in the leg. The pain is greater than might be expected, even when the limb is immobilised. It is relentless in character, and often not greatly relieved by opiates. The limb is tense and swollen, and there may be induration (a late sign) over the affected compartment. Tenderness is diffuse, and can be elicited some distance from the fracture itself. There is pain on passive stretching of the muscles arising in the affected compartment (e.g. by passive movement of the foot or toes), and there may be muscle paralysis. There may be complaint of sensory disturbance in the leg or foot and this may be confirmed clinically; loss of vibration sense is an early finding. The distal pulses may be reduced or absent.

The intercompartmental pressures may be monitored; this should be done as close to the fracture as possible. A differential tissue pressure (the diastolic blood pressure minus the intracompartment's pressure) below 30mm of Hg is an indication for surgery.

TREATMENT

Prophylaxis Where there is an open fracture with extensive muscle damage, the compartment involved should be widely decompressed at the time of the initial exploration.

Established cases Prompt decompression of *all four compartments* is advised. This is generally best performed through two 'safe' incisions (see following frames for details). (A single lateral incision can give access, but the dissection can be difficult; it is best reserved for cases where there is concurrent damage to the anterior tibial artery, when the viability of the intervening skin bridge might be in doubt.)

Aftercare Often one of the two wounds may be closed directly, and the other by controlled tension or split skin grafting. If the swelling is marked, both should be left open; then, in most cases, both may be closed after 3–5 days when the swelling has decreased; skin grafting is rarely required.

57. The safe incisions: These are designed to avoid the perforating arteries, and should be used for compartment decompressions or to extend existing wounds, especially if fasciocutaneous flaps are going to be required. The anterolateral (a) should be placed 2 cm lateral to the anterior border of the tibia. The medial (m) is made 1–2 cm posterior to the medial border of the tibia. In both cases the incisions are made straight through skin and fascia.

58. Anterior and peroneal compartment decompression: Use a 15 cm 'safe' anterolateral incision. Grasp the investing fascia forming the roof of the antero-lateral compartment with Köcher forceps to keep it under tension, and split it longitudinally with blunt scissors – aiming proximally for the patella and distally for the mid-point of the ankle. Then retract the lateral skin flap and divide the anterior peroneal septum to decompress the lateral (peroneal) compartment. (ac = anterior compartment; lc = lateral compartment. Fascia shown in dark grey.)

59. Decompression of posterior compartments: Use a 15 cm 'safe' medial incision in the distal part of the leg to open the superficial posterior compartment. Then, to open the deep compartment, separate the soleus from its tibial attachments: begin distally where its tendinous part blends with gastrocnemius, and working proximally detach the soleal bridge from the tibia. Finally the fascial coverings of the three deep bi-pennate muscles may be divided. (s = soleus; g = gastrocnemius; tp = tibialis posterior)

TIBIA/FIBULA, *Diaphyseal Segment : 42–*

60. AO Classification of fractures of the tibia/fibula, diaphyseal segment (42–):

Type A fractures are simple fractures.
A1 = Spiral: .1 fibula intact; .2 fibula fractured at another level; .3 fibula fractured at the same level.
A2 = Oblique fracture (30° or more): .1 fibula intact; .2 fibula fractured at another level; .3 fibula fractured at the same level.
A3 = Transverse fracture (less than 30° of obliquity): .1 fibula intact; .2 fibula fractured at another level; .3 fibula fractured at the same level.

Type B fractures are wedge fractures.
B1 = Spiral: .1 fibula intact; .2 fibula fractured at another level; .3 fibula fractured at the same level.
B2 = Bending wedge fracture: .1 fibula intact; .2 fibula fractured at another level; .3 fibula fractured at the same level.
B3 = Fragmented wedge: .1 fibula intact; .2 fibula fractured at another level; .3 fibula fractured at the same level.

Type C fractures are complex fractures.
C1 = Spiral: .1 with two intermediate fragments; .2 with three intermediate fragments; .3 with more than three intermediate fragments.
C2 = Segmental: .1 with one intermediate segment; .2 with an intermediate segment and additional wedge; .3 with two intermediate segments.
C3 = Irregular: .1 with two or three intermediate fragments; .2 with shattering over a length of less than 4 cm; .3 with shattering over a length of 4 cm or more.

SELF-TEST

61. What complication has occurred in this uniting fracture of the tibia in the distal third?

62. What pattern of fracture is present? How is it being treated?

63. What complication is present in this united tibial fracture? What effect will this have?

64. What is being treated here at present, and what earlier treatment was employed?

65. What complication is shown in this radiograph of a tibial fracture?

66. These radiographs were taken through plaster 10 weeks after injury. Describe the fracture. What further treatment would you advocate? What is the prognosis?

67. What does this radiograph show?

ANSWERS TO SELF-TEST

61. The radiograph shows the disturbance of bone trabeculation typical of Sudeck's atrophy (complex regional pain syndrome).

62. This shows a spiral fracture of the tibia at the junction of the mid and distal thirds being treated in plaster. The position in this *single* view appears excellent. AO = 42–A1.1.

63. Mal-union of the fracture is present with lateral angulation. The plane of the ankle joint is affected, and secondary, degenerative arthritis in it is possible.

64. There is a fracture of the mid-shaft of the tibia, with an associated malleolar injury. The former is being treated with a locked medullary nail, and the latter with cross screws. The fracture was an open one, and treated originally with an external fixator, the bone scars of the threaded pins being still visible.

65. Hypertrophic non-union is present. AO = 42–A3.1.

66. The radiographs are of an oblique fracture of the tibia in the middle third, with an associated fibular fracture at the junction of the middle and lower thirds. Both fractures are uniting, and bridging callus is well formed. The general alignment is good. No correction at this late stage is required: the patient will require to continue with fixation for about another 4 weeks before plaster can be discarded (or a cast brace may be substituted). There will be approximately 1 cm of shortening, but the functional prognosis is excellent. AO = 42–A2.2.

67. There has been a largely transverse fracture of the tibia at the junction of the proximal and middle thirds, and this has been treated with a T2™ nail. Locking screws have been inserted both proximally and distally. There is a disturbance of bone texture in the proximal two-thirds typical of Paget's disease, and there was in the lateral view an associated anterior curvature of the bone of sabre pattern. At the time of surgery the fracture was exposed and a wedge of bone (with its apex placed posteriorly) excised in order to correct the deformity and facilitate the nailing. AO = 42–A3.3

101. Ankle dislocation without fracture: Rarely the ankle may dislocate without fracture. Although rupture of both medial and lateral ligaments must take place, conservative management by closed manipulative reduction and plaster fixation may achieve a good result, although some prefer surgical repair. Avascular necrosis of the talus is a minor risk in this situation.

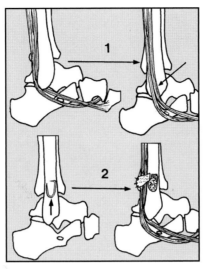

102. Recurrent dislocation of peroneal tendons: This is a rare condition in which eversion causes painful clicking sensations as the peroneal tendons repeatedly snap over the lateral malleolus (1). The condition is associated with a defect in the superior peroneal retinaculum. A flap of bone and periosteum can be used to reconstruct the defective ligament (2).

103. Footballer's ankle and osteochondritis tali: Tibial and/or talar osteophytes (1) may arise in footballers from repeated anterior capsular tears, and limit dorsiflexion. Excision for this is seldom indicated, but if symptoms are commanding arthroscopic debridement may be tried. Pain may follow a fresh tear (treat symptomatically by POP fixation) or from early ankle joint osteoarthritis. For osteochondritis tali (2), see p. 409.

104. Complications of ankle injuries: Swelling: Swelling persisting for weeks or even months after fixation has been discarded is so common as to be an almost normal occurrence. Assuming that the fracture has united in a good position, local supportive measures should be continued until resolution. The patient should be reassured and advised regarding elevation and activity.

105. Complex regional pain syndrome/ Sudeck's atrophy: Where swelling is gross, and especially if the toes are involved, suspect Sudeck's atrophy. There may be glazing of the skin and pain. Radiographs may show typical porotic changes, and confirm union of the fracture. Intensive physiotherapy, continued use of supports and other measures may be required (see also p. 100). Convalescence may be expected to be slow with occasionally some permanent functional impairment.

106. Stiffness, 'weakness' and disturbance of gait: Again, assuming sound union, these symptoms generally respond rapidly to appropriate physiotherapy and occupational therapy. Progress may be assessed by charting the range of ankle joint movements. (The normal range is indicated in the illustration, but compare the sides.) Note also the range in the subtalar joint.

107. Instability: Instability due to lateral ligament damage has been described (see Frame 95 et seq). Instability may also follow damage to the medial structures. Non-union of a large medial malleolar fragment should be treated by internal fixation: additional bone grafting may be necessary (1). When the tip only is involved, it may be excised and the lateral ligament sutured to the stump (2).

108. Osteoarthritis (a): Considering the incidence of ankle fractures, osteoarthritis is an uncommon complication. It is most likely to follow compression fractures, and fractures with residual diastasis or talotibial incongruity. Note in this example of an old compression fracture the central split in the tibial surface, the broadening of the mortise and the narrowed joint space.

109. Osteoarthritis (b): If symptoms of pain, swelling, stiffness and disturbance of gait are troublesome, then fusion may be advised. In the Crawford–Adams fusion, the articular surfaces are cleared, the fibula is inlaid in the talus and tibia and held in position with cross screws. Late function is generally good due to persistent midtarsal movement.

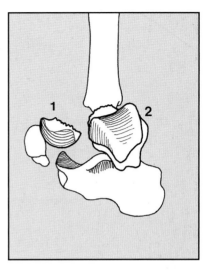

7. Classification (d): *Group III injuries:* With further dorsiflexion and upward force (1) the tibia is driven between the two talar fragments. The posterior fragment is extruded backwards, while at the same time the convex posterior articular surface of the calcaneus (2) guides it medially. It comes to rest with its medial surface (3) caught on the sustentaculum tali (4).

8. Classification (e): In its final position (*ctd*) the main portion of the talus lies on the medial side of the ankle, with its fractured surface (5) pointing laterally. All three sources of blood supply are disturbed. The risks of avascular necrosis are high, rising to 85%.

9. Classification (f): In the rare *Group IV injury*, the head of the talus dislocates from the navicular (1) in association with a Group III (2) or a Group II injury. The incidence of avascular necrosis here is also high.

10. Diagnosis: The diagnosis may be suspected from the history, but is made radiologically. Care must be taken to differentiate between Type 1 and Type 2 injuries. If doubt exists, two laterals, one in dorsiflexion (1) and one in plantar flexion (2) should be taken and compared. These will reveal any subluxation (Type 2 illustrated).

11. Treatment of Type I injuries: Apply a padded plaster with a toe platform and elevate for about a week (1). Then non-weight bearing with crutches for 3 months (2). The fracture is then assessed out of plaster for union and absence of avascular necrosis (3). If there are no complications, weight bearing may commence with a light support (4). Physiotherapy will be required for the ankle, subtalar joint and calf.

12. Treatment of Type II injuries (a): While some prefer open reduction for all these fractures, closed methods may be attempted: (1) The foot is plantar flexed and everted. (2) A padded plaster is applied in this position and check radiographs taken. If a satisfactory reduction has been obtained, then conservative treatment may be continued.

13. Treatment of Type II injuries (b): (3) The limb is elevated for a week before (4) non-weight bearing is permitted. After 3–4 weeks the plaster is changed under intensifier control and the foot brought up to a right angle (5). Non-weight bearing is continued for a further 6 weeks. Thereafter, if the fracture is united and there is no evidence of avascular necrosis, weight bearing may be allowed with support (6). Physiotherapy will almost certainly be required.

14. Treatment of Group II injuries (c): If closed methods fail in obtaining a reduction, open reduction will be required. The fracture may be secured with a Kirschner wire passed backwards from the head of the talus into the body, with the aftercare being similar to that described in the previous frame.
The Kirschner wire may be removed at the change of plaster. For more rigid fixation, a cannulated screw may be preferred.

15. Treatment of Group III injuries (a): The displaced portion of the talus is situated subcutaneously, and there should be no delay in reducing it as the overlying skin is tightly stretched over the bone and likely to slough. Facilities for open reduction should be available, but closed methods may be attempted first. Begin by gripping the heel and applying traction to it.

the head (5). Cannulated screws may also be used; these can be threaded over Kirschner wires which have been inserted temporarily to hold the reduction (6). The AO group, with an eye to rapid mobilisation, in fact recommend internal fixation along these lines for all talar neck fractures.
Treatment of Group IV injuries: These uncommon injuries are likely to require open reduction. All fragments should be retained, even if completely detached and obviously avascular. On no account should the talus be excised.

Complications of talar neck fractures (a):
Skin necrosis: The skin may become tightly stretched over a displaced talus and undergo necrosis with late sloughing. *Early reduction is imperative to avoid this complication.*

(b): Open injuries: Thorough debridement of the wound is essential, but again every effort must be made to retain the main fragments. Treatment should follow the usual lines established for the management of open fractures. If sepsis occurs *in conjunction with avascular necrosis*, healing may be obtained only after excision of the avascular fragments.

16. Treatment of Group III injuries (b): Maintaining traction (1), use the knee (2) to dorsiflex the foot. Pull the heel slightly forward and evert it (3) to open up the space for the talus. Apply strong pressure over the displaced body of the talus (4), pressing laterally, but also slightly anteriorly and downwards. Now plantar flex the foot. If purchase on the heel is poor, a Steinman pin through the heel and a calliper may be used.

17. Treatment of Group III injuries (c): After reduction, proceed with elevation and gradual mobilisation as described in Frame 13 above. If closed reduction fails (as it often does), open reduction will be necessary. The condition of the skin and any planned internal fixation will dictate the incision(s). These fractures may be fixed (best through a posterolateral incision) with one or two cancellous screws passed from behind through the body of the talus and into

SELF-TEST

108. What is this injury? What complication is likely to develop?

109. What abnormalities are shown on this radiograph?

110. What is this injury? What treatment would be advised?

111. Describe this radiograph of a crushed foot. What would be the main principles of treatment?

112. What injuries have been dealt with in this case of polytrauma?

ANSWERS TO SELF-TEST

108. Type III fracture of the neck of the talus. The incidence of avascular necrosis in this type of injury approximates to 85%.

109. There is an undisplaced fracture of the anterior process of the calcaneus as a result of recent trauma. In addition there is a small avulsion fracture of the dorsal aspect of the navicular, probably of long standing.

110. Tarsometatarsal dislocation: if a recent injury, open reduction would be advised; if an old injury, surgical wedge correction with a tarsometatarsal fusion might be indicated.

111. Comminuted fracture of the first metatarsal. Fractures of the shafts of the 2nd and 3rd metatarsals. Double fracture of the 4th metatarsal. Fracture of the neck of the 5th metatarsal. Lateral

displacement. The injury is open (horizontal streaks of ingrained dirt can be seen). Treatment: if the foot is viable, 1. Debridement. 2. Reduction and Kirschner wire fixation of at least the 1st and 2nd metatarsals. 3. Plaster back shell or split padded plaster, elevation, observation, compartment pressure monitoring, infection prophylaxis (including antitetanus), etc.

112. There has been a bi-malleolar fracture of the ankle which has been dealt with by plating and screwing of the fibula; and a fracture of the medial malleolus has been held with two screws. There has been a fracture of the neck of the talus which has been reduced and held with two Acutrak screws. Just off the film there is a fracture of the base of the 5th metatarsal, also held with an Acutrak screw.

The organisation and running of fracture clinics varies from hospital to hospital. These differences are often dictated by the layout of the departments involved – records, appointments, secretarial, clinical, treatment, plaster, theatre and X-ray – and and also by an established line of practice. A system which has worked for a number of years is difficult to change, as an apparently obvious improvement in one area may upset the smooth running of others – to the overall detriment; and change of any kind in an established system is unusual if it attracts universal acceptance. Those who work in fracture clinics have usually to do so within a framework imposed upon them, and it would be invidious to suggest a 'best way' of doing things. Nevertheless it might be helpful for the beginner who is confronted for the first time with a fracture clinic to offer a few guidelines on the handling of the actual consultation.

The newcomer to a fracture clinic is usually impressed by the number of cases dealt with in a short space of time. This speed often conceals the number of rather important decisions that are made about the patients' care. These decisions are, of course, determined by the basic principles of fracture treatment, but to ensure the smooth running of the clinic, the most professional and kindliest contact with the patient, and the avoidance of any error in management, the use of a simple system, at least at the beginning, may be of some help.

Assuming that the usual courtesies of greeting have been made, each consultation should start with asking the two questions – 'what?' and 'when?' and end with asking 'when?' and 'what?'. In the middle there are a number of things to go through which can be conveniently dealt with under three headings, each starting with the letter A – 'the three As'.

THE FRACTURE CONSULTATION

'WHAT?'

Every decision that is made, and everything that is done, is directly dependent on the diagnosis. *This must be clearly stated at the beginning of the notes on the first fracture clinic attendance,* where they will serve as a guide to everyone who sees the patient subsequently. It is a never-ending source of astonishment as to how difficult it may be to find this information, the time taken often varying directly in proportion to the size of the records. If there is a problem, a glance at the initial radiographs (they alone are helpful to label) may give the answer. Time spent establishing the diagnosis is essential. Recording it will prevent the effort having to be repeated at the patient's next attendance.

'WHEN?'

The point here is to establish the time that has passed since the patient's injury. While this can obviously be calculated on every occasion from the entries made on the day of injury and on the clinic visit, it is of greater practical value to give the elapsed time.

It is more professional to establish these primary facts before confronting the patient, rather than searching through the notes in his presence. When making the appropriate notes, where brevity should not compromise accuracy, the addition of a qualifier in the case of the diagnosis may be helpful: e.g.:

correct. A check radiograph taken after application of the plaster shows the fracture in anatomical position, and there is no talar shift.

The notes record that he was seen the day following the injury and the circulation was thought to be satisfactory. On his present attendance the toes are noted to be a little swollen, and he is complaining of pain in the little toe which is concealed by the cast that extends over it. This area must be inspected, and the excess plaster is trimmed back exposing the toe. Although the toe is red, it is judged that the relief of local pressure will allow a rapid return to normal. The degree of swelling of the toes suggests that it might be unwise to permit weight bearing at this stage.

The patient is told that although his fracture is in an excellent position, as is commonly the case, he has too much swelling to allow him to take weight as yet through his plaster. He is advised to continue using his crutches, and to elevate the limb whenever possible. He is encouraged to exercise the toes.

His job is found to be that of a representative, and involves a mixture of driving, walking and sitting. He is advised that he will have to remain in a plaster cast for 6–8 weeks, and that while in his plaster he should not attempt to drive. Considering the nature of his job which cannot be adjusted to suit his circumstances, he must expect to be absent for at least 2 months. His actual time off will depend on his progress after coming out of plaster, but there is a good chance of his being able to get back to his particular job within 3 months of the injury.

His notes might read:

4/7 since # R lat. mall. POP trimmed. See 2/52 ? heel.

On his second fracture clinic appointment the toe swelling has subsided. The plaster is checked for slackness, and considered to be still offering adequate support. It is noted that the sole of the plaster is a little soft as a result of some weight having been put on it. The upper end of the cast at the back is a little high and is restricting knee flexion. The sole is reinforced, the calf of the plaster trimmed, and a walking heel or boot applied.

The patient is told that he may now start taking full weight through the limb; but that to begin with he should use his crutches until he has gained confidence, when he may or may not feel the need to use a single walking stick. He is asked to return in 4 weeks when it will be decided whether he can come out of plaster, or whether a short further period of plaster fixation will be needed. He is also advised to return in the interim if he has any problem with his plaster.

The note may read:

2/52. Sole reinforced. Heel. See 4/52 POP off and X-ray ankle on arrival.

On his third attendance the limb is inspected out of plaster. There is no swelling, and no tenderness in the region of the fracture. A check radiograph (which some would regard as being optional) shows some early callus formation in the region of the fracture whose position has been maintained. Movements of the ankle are restricted to 5° dorsiflexion and 10° plantar flexion.

Union of the fracture is assessed as being sufficient for the patient to remain out of plaster. It is anticipated that as he mobilises the ankle there will be some swelling, and he is given a Tubigrip or crepe bandage support. It is thought that he will rapidly regain most of his ankle and foot movements, and that although the need for physiotherapy will have to be kept in mind, this will probably not be required. He is shown how to exercise the foot and ankle on his own.

The patient is told that his fracture is progressing very well, but that he is likely to develop some rather persistent swelling of his ankle. The support he has been given to counteract this should be removed when in bed at night. He is advised to return in 2 weeks' time when he will be assessed regarding the need for further treatment or when he can return to work.

The note may read:

6/52. POP off. # uniting. Tubigrip. See 2/52 ? physio. ? discharge.

On his fourth visit a trace of swelling is noted, but he has recovered all but the last 5° of plantar flexion in the ankle, and foot movements are full. He has no complaint of pain and says he is anxious to return to work which he now thinks he will be able to manage. He wonders when he might return to playing golf and squash.

As he has no pain in the ankle and has recovered a good range of movements, no physiotherapy is necessary and it should be safe for him to drive and try going back to work. He is advised to continue wearing his support until any tendency to swelling has disappeared.

The presence of some swelling suggests that it would be wise not to overdo his weight-bearing activities. A reasonable approach might be to recommend that after a further 2 weeks he might try a half round of golf, and be guided by any subsequent discomfort and swelling. As far as squash is concerned, where stress on the ankles is particularly high, it would be advisable to defer this until a full 3 months from the time of the original injury, and until all swelling of the ankle has subsided.

He should be told that at this stage, in view of his progress and the anticipation of a full recovery, that there is no immediate need for him to reattend. Should, however, he become unhappy about his progress then he should make a review appointment. It should be mentioned that his doctor will be sent a letter with a summary of the history, present findings and recommendations.

The final note then need only be '**See discharge letter'.** The discharge letter itself need not be long, but should cover the main points in the history, the diagnosis, the treatment, and the prognosis. Such a letter might read:

'Mr _____ attended the Casualty Department on ____ with an undis-placed fracture of the right lateral malleolus sustained in a fall down some steps. It was treated by 6 weeks' fixation in POP and it has united in good position. He has regained a good range of movements in the ankle, but he has still a little swelling. He can now return to work, but should avoid contact sports for a further month at least. He has been discharged today, but I have advised him to return should he have any problem.'

Enjoy your clinics!